S0-ABQ-094

Million Ways to Live

6 Principles for Your Lifestyle Transformation

Luke Sniewski

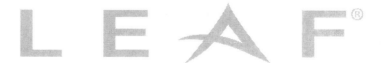

Copyright © 2014 LEAF Lifestyle, Inc.

All rights reserved.

www.leaflifestyle.com

www.lukesniewski.com

ISBN: 978-0-9899111-3-9

This book is dedicated to all the health professionals and healers who empower the individuals they work with to be their own wellness guru. Health is a personal responsibility we must all have the courage to shoulder. Cheers to those who impart that wisdom onto others and provide them with the necessary education, mentoring and guidance. Keep fighting the good fight.

TABLE OF CONTENTS

To my best friend, muse, partner in crime and best mom Jack could ever ask for, Claire. Can't wait for our next adventure.

A special thanks to Lenny for teaching me how to use my own brain and Graham for teaching me how to turn it off.

Lastly, thank you to all those who let me experiment my theories and methods on them. Without you, this book wouldn't be possible.

To Lenny Parracino, Graham Mead, Philip Ackerman-Leist, David Diaz, Tanner Martty, Troy Alvarado, Phong Starzewski, Shimi Minhas, John Brown, Dhru Purohit, Jill Miller, Robert Faust, Chelsea Roff, Robert Picard, John Berardi, Michael Brown, Bruce Lipton, Chris Miller, Seth Casden, Mike Mahler, Vince Guagliano, David Tabain, Mark Morgan, Martin Sniewski, Francis Rosignolo, Fritjof Capra, Daniel Quinn, Damian Rosochacki, Nicholas Davey, Zero Kazama, Darin Fujimori, Jeffery Bomberger, Tim Ferriss, Joselynne Boschen, Sergio Gonzales, Kelley Coughlan, Preston Clarke, Danael Karlsson, Jerome Mercier, Carol Cotner Thompson, Cory Weiss, Christopher Rivas, Serge Gracovetsky, Frank Forencich, Daniel Lieberman, Judy Delany and many many others, whether knowingly or unknowingly, you have served as my mentors, guides, teachers and motivators over the years.
Thank you.

Preface

"As to methods there may be a million and then some, but principles are few.
Those who grasp principles can successfully select their own methods. Those
who try methods, ignoring principles, are sure to have trouble."
– Ralph Waldo Emerson

"Everything has been figured out, except how to live." – Jean-Paul Sartre

The most dangerous job I've had: Certified Public Accountant. I'd spent many years before that playing football, a career that included playing quarterback professionally for the Italian Football League. I was knocked down and tackled on a consistent basis by 250-pound players. Thankfully, I didn't end up with permanent injuries. In my post-football years I thought life within the four walls of a cubicle would be safe. It turns out sitting in my comfortable chair at my desk turned out to be worse for my health than the speeding rush of linebackers and defensive ends.

Within just a few months at my first accounting job, I noticed pains in my body that I'd never felt before. Neck pain, throbbing in my lower back, elbow tingling, numbness in my wrist … My new 'injuries' just didn't make sense. *Were these just past football injuries reemerging?* I decided to do my own research. It turns out sitting down is really bad for your health. Like, *really* bad. It's safe to say that what I learned in the first week of research served as all the motivation I needed to leave a promising and stable accounting career behind and pursue a career in the health and wellness industry instead.

When the average person visits a doctor, it's normally only when they're sick. When they visit a physical therapist, it's normally only when they're injured. We generally book appointments to see medical professionals to either make sure we're on the right path or when we're hurt and need fixing. I consider it complete luck and good fortune, then, that I began my health and wellness career as a personal trainer.

As a personal trainer, I often saw my clients two to five times a week. The contact hours I had with clients provided invaluable educational experiences that could never be replicated in a classroom or by reading textbooks and studies. My clients were, have been and always will be my best teachers. The most important lesson that personal training has taught me is that there is no such thing as a magic workout. In fact, after being repeatedly humbled in my early training years, I realized I needed to know more—*a lot* more—if I wanted to help more people with their overall health and wellbeing.

In short, understanding exercise science wasn't enough. There's so much more to healthy living than just a 'kick ass' workout, though my inner jock fought this notion tooth-and-nail. Changing someone's life means teaching—or rather *re-teaching*— a person *how to live*. It's their total daily lifestyle that matters, not just one portion of it. The way a person eats, moves, laughs, loves, communicates, learns, thinks and feels all contribute to their overall health. Everything counts. It seems like common sense, but it fails the test of common practice.

So I chose nutrition as my next educational challenge. I traveled all over the country, learning from the best minds in the industry en route to becoming a Certified Nutritionist, which improved my ability to help people with their health. After all, *food is thy medicine and medicine thy food*. I helped more people with greater effect, but it wasn't enough. Diet and exercise are important, but so are tissue quality, posture and flexibility. That's why I became a Certified Neuromuscular Therapist too. Working with trigger points and damaged muscle tissue opened up a whole new world of pain-free movement my clients had never experienced. It still wasn't enough, though. I went to cooking school in order to practically teach my clients about how to control their food quality. Finally, I earned my Masters of Science in Sustainable Food Systems. Understanding the food production systems responsible for the entire nation's food supply proved to be an educational endeavor that connected even more dots. When you consider the social, political, economic, environmental and technological components of this country's food system, you can easily discern what is marketing hype and what is substantive knowledge. More importantly, you gain a broader understanding of our nation's obesity and chronic disease epidemics.

I've learned from countless books, clients, case studies, articles, mentors and doctors—and it's amazing how many different opinions there are out there. It's no wonder, then, that many people have absolutely no idea where to turn for health information. But during my journey through informational chaos, I learned that the most important teacher was and always will be *myself*. Living everything I preached, experimenting on myself and often times on my clients, I learned through trial and error something far more important than what methods and practices work for optimizing health. I learned *why* and *how*, which are both infinitely more important than blindly following *what* to do. I wanted the fundamental truths; simplicity in a world of chaos.

I concluded that there are six fundamental principles of healthy living, which you'll learn in just a few moments. These six principles have provided me with an amazing filter for health information that finds its way into my mental landscape. For example, if I read or hear about something that contradicts these principles, then I proceed with a healthy amount of skepticism and investigate further. Clever advertising and less-than-healthy fads are easily identified when armed with these six Healthy Lifestyle Principles. Conversely, if it's supported by the principles, then it's likely to be a healthy option worth exploring or experimenting with. After all, our world is full of so many healthy traditions and ways of life, it would be shame not to try as many as possible.

Million Ways to Live is about sharing the knowledge that has allowed me to help countless numbers of friends, clients, family members, loved ones and perfect strangers. The main reason why these methods have worked is because they empower people to listen to their own bodies and discover what works best for them— because there's no one right way to peak health and wellness. Optimal health is gained only after personal empowerment. It's a journey of self-discovery—one I hope the reader will take with the help of this book.

That's why I wrote this book. I know that the lessons I've learned can help anyone, regardless of their fitness and health goals. Why? Because there's a certain simplicity when it comes to healthy living that's often difficult to see amid the cluttered landscape of marketing hype and fads. But by simply following these principles, any health and fitness goal is possible.

The lessons in this book have helped my clients get on the cover of Men's Health Magazine, lose an astonishing 100 pounds in six months (and keep it off), and achieve health they never thought possible. One of my favorite moments with a client is when they suddenly realize that they haven't been sick since starting their program. A strengthened and resilient immune system is just one of the many benefits of a new and improved healthy lifestyle. The six principles in this book are universal and can help you to with your very own Lifestyle Transformation.

Structure of *Million Ways to Live*

The introduction to this book discusses why the process of becoming overweight and obese is inherently rooted in your everyday lifestyle, or the way in which you live your life day to day. Why is weight discussed? Because it's one of the few obvious, visible, quantitative and measurable variables that we can use to assess whether your attempt at trying to become healthy is actually working. Since obesity is correlated with so many chronic diseases—and because we are in the midst of an obesity epidemic—the implication is that gaining weight is unhealthy while losing weight is healthy for our bodies and our economy.

The remaining core chapters of the book are devoted to the six Healthy Lifestyle Principles: **Real Food, Movement, Rest & Relaxation, Lifelong Learning, Community and Love**. These simple, universal principles can be used to accurately describe the lives of healthy people around the world for millennia. These principles are rooted in basic and fundamental human *needs* (determined by nature and natural law), rather than trivial *wants* like six-pack abs or a perkier butt (determined by magazines and advertisers). We need real food, daily movement, ample rest, creativity and learning, a supportive community and love in order to thrive. When you provide your body with what it needs, your body, mind and spirit will in turn thrive.

Regardless of which school of thought or wellness philosophy you research, you will find that these six principles consistently pop up. It's what everyone universally agrees upon, yet what only a few have a practical knowledge of. We know this stuff, but we just don't practice it. We're confused, lost and—worse of all—defensive and closed-minded. This is the direct result of living in a world of infinite information without appropriate filters and guidelines to use it. The magic is in the application of knowledge.

To say there's a general lack of trust in the health and wellness world would be an understatement.

These six Healthy Lifestyle Principles will give you some much-needed confidence to not only find health for yourself, but also remain open-minded and accepting of other ways of healthy living. There's so much in this world to try, experiment with and enjoy. Keep yourself open to possibility, in order to learn more about the world and yourself.

Once you learn the six Healthy Lifestyle Principles, you can apply them into your life in many different ways and combinations. It all depends on your personality, physiology, culture, fitness level and, most importantly, your individual goals. That's why this book is called *Million Ways to Live*. Even though there are six Healthy Lifestyle Principles, they can be applied in numerous—millions of—ways. We live in a globalized world and therefore have an endless supply of options virtually on tap that are invaluable to our personal growth and development.

Because every person is unique in their own way, *Million Ways to Live* provides a framework for self-exploration and self-discovery, something that's essential for achieving optimal health. No one knows your body better than you. So in essence, this book provides a blueprint for a healthy life. Then, once you've built the foundation provided by the blueprint, it's up to you how you decorate it with your personal finishing touches. Your healthy lifestyle will become the creative expression of your inner being—your true authentic self.

The chapters in this book are standalone compositions that can be read separately without impacting your understanding of the rest of the book, so feel free to jump to the chapter that focuses on the Healthy Lifestyle Principle you need the most help with if you don't want to read the book from start to finish. It may make more sense to start with the principle you need the most help with, since addressing the weakest link of your lifestyle will undoubtedly impact your life the most. If you know your diet is your greatest downfall, start with the Real Food chapter. If you already follow a structured and successful exercise and nutrition plan, but have an incessantly negative voice in your head that makes you depressed, anxious or angry, you'll probably create the most positive impact on your life by jumping to the Love chapter. Mix and match the Healthy Lifestyle Principles until your own lifestyle has been transformed the way that works for you.

Each chapter begins with a story of common issues, pitfalls and thought processes many people plunge into when attempting to become healthier. They follow a fictional character named David as he begins his journey towards his own health and wellness. David knows it's easy to get confused by the big wide world of healthy living—he's been there too. That's why his stories may sound familiar; they focus on the common mistakes people make when they embark on their own lifestyle transformation programs. These narratives will resonate with you.

Each chapter then provides a thorough outline of each principle, so you can directly apply the lessons to your own life and understand why it contributes to a healthy lifestyle. Finally, at the conclusion of every chapter is a practical application section designed to get you started on your own path to healthy living. The tips presented in the *Healthy Habits* section of each chapter are your jump-start towards healthier living.

Lastly, this book is grounded and based on what I believe to be common sense, age-old tradition that's been around for centuries, and real results by real people. That being said, it also includes plenty of citations from scientific and academic journals to satisfy the palates of healthy skeptics. But the truth is that, if the citations and sources were to be stripped from the following pages, this book would still rest upon a firm foundation of common sense and, more importantly, historically common practices that have simply been forgotten in the clutter of the modern world.

It's important to note that the recommendations provided in *Million Ways to Live* are intentionally centered on habits. When people take steps towards their goals, they will undoubtedly face behaviors, programming and bad habits from their past which have prevented them from reaching their goals many times before. By focusing on changing habits, you will work towards changing your in-built programming, and stop those bad habits that have incessantly thwarted your attempts at healthy living over and over again in the past. When you integrate sustainable habits into your daily life, you set yourself up for a lifetime of health.

I promise I won't leave you out in the cold when you finish reading the book, though. Your own healthy lifestyle is made easy with an easy-to-follow 52-week program called Lifestyle Transformation, located at the end of the book. This year-long program takes you through all 26 habits from the book in a structured, mindful and sustainable way—one habit at a time, so it's not too daunting. Focus 100% of your energy on the single habit being practiced and follow it through every day. If you dedicate two weeks to every habit, by the end of the year you will have an entirely new lifestyle—one that's grounded in health and wellness. Your leaner, fitter and healthier body will provide all the evidence you need to confirm the success of your physical, mental and emotional transformation.

So only one question remains:

Are you ready for *your* Lifestyle Transformation?

Five Goals for Readers

"You can learn to follow the inner self, the inner physician that tells you where to go. Healing is simply attempting to do more of those things that bring joy and fewer of those things that bring pain." – O. Carl Simonton

"If man is to survive, he will have learned to take a delight in the essential differences between men and between cultures. He will learn that differences in ideas and attitudes are a delight, part of life's exciting variety, not something to fear." – Gene Roddenberry

Bucket lists are typically filled with dreams of traveling the world, climbing mountains, completing marathons or meeting famous people. But the number one item on my bucket list is to positively impact the lives of one million people. I hope this book can be a step in the right direction since its fundamental purpose is to help people with the most important part of their life: their personal health. Here are five goals I hope every reader will reach as a result of reading this book.

1. Create a Blueprint for a Healthy Lifestyle

The first and obvious purpose of this book is to teach people how to improve their physical, mental and emotional health. The six principles discussed in *Million Ways to Live* should set the foundation for life-long healthy living. They are, of course, meant to be adapted in your own unique way because there's no one quite like you in every single way. Choose how to apply these principles to your own lives based on the many variables that make you truly unique. We all have differences in physiology, faith, culture, personality, fitness goals and social networks, just to name a few.

Regardless of one's individuality, though, the common thread uniting every single reader is the six Healthy Lifestyle Principles and their role in helping you regain control of your life. Making yourself consciously aware of your lifestyle and concurrently focusing on your wellbeing is the first step to taking back control of your health. This book is your introduction to the healthy life you deserve as your birthright.

2. Thrive, Don't Just Survive

Your body is incredibly resilient. Just look around you. It's easy to see how unhealthy people can be, yet they continue to function on a daily basis. The truth is that the human body can survive a lifetime of junk food, smoking and a host of other unhealthy habits, because unhealthy habits don't cause instant death. Instead, they cause a slow, torturous and numbing death; that's why they're called *chronic* diseases. The path to death is so slow and almost invisible that we have plenty of time—a lifetime, sometimes—to adjust to our lowered states of living, actually accepting them as normal. A perpetual decline in health after adolescence has almost come to be expected.

This is something I refuse to accept and believe. That is why *Million Ways to Live* is not simply about surviving. It's about thriving. It's about implementing a Lifestyle Transformation aimed at substituting unhealthy habits that destroy your body with healthy habits that build lifelong health. It's about feeling and experiencing the vibrancy of what life is meant to feel like, when you satisfy fundamental human needs rather than short-term bursts of perceived satisfaction derived from materialism and consumerism.

3. Become Your Own Wellness Guru

Healthy living is an individual journey, not a final destination. On your journey towards optimal health and wellness, experience is the best teacher. Experiment on yourself. The contents of this book provide a foundation for your life. Where you take the knowledge and how you apply it will depend on your personal goals and how your experience unfolds.

The bottom line is that you will become your own teacher. You will explore different schools of thoughts, ideas and methods to see which ones work best for you and your body. Listen to your body; it's your best teacher. Keep the strategies that work for you; discard the rest. *Million Ways to Live* will be an education in connecting with the innate wisdom of your body and understanding what it needs to thrive. You will become your own wellness guru.

4. Develop an Attitude of Acceptance

The role of a great healer is to solve, lead and inspire, never to judge, condemn or frighten. Avoid negativity and judgment, and use empathy and open dialogue instead to succeed in your own lifestyle transformation. Inspire health by living an inspiring life. Remain open-minded throughout the process because there is no one right way to live. There never has been, and there never will be.

Lead by example. Don't try to fear, bully, patronize and hurt people. You'll find that you actually have more in common with the people you disagree with than you first realize. As the title of this book suggests, there are a million ways to live, not just one. Understanding and accepting the viewpoints of others will help you on your own path to optimal health and wellness.

5. Eat for All Humankind

When I first chose to eat organic food, it was largely for selfish reasons—my own health. But as I continued to learn and dig deeper, I realized my consumption and lifestyle decisions impact not only my own life, but the lives of the people around me. It was a strange awakening when I realized that the money I use to buy food products actually casts a vote for which companies, agricultural processes and laborers are ultimately responsible for my overall wellbeing.

Not only do these decisions impact my life, but they impact the life of my son, Jack. If I can do one thing to help the next generation, it is to support those business and agricultural practices that work with—rather than exploit—the natural environment. These connections and correlations never existed to me before I started focusing my life on health. Then I realized that personal health is intimately linked with environmental health. What's good for the planet is good for us. That's why the conclusion of *Million Ways to Live* discusses sustainability and how our daily lifestyle decisions impact the world around us. The decisions you make today impact the future in more ways than you know. So choose wisely.

Introduction: Meet David

"The greatest miracle on Earth is the human body. It is stronger and wiser than you may realize, and improving its ability to self-heal is within your control."
– Dr Fabrizio Mancini

"Health is a state of complete harmony of the body, mind and spirit. When one is free from physical disabilities and mental distractions, the gates of the soul open." – B.K.S. Iyengar

"Three … Two … One … Happy New Year!" Champagne pops, glasses clink, cheering erupts and colorful confetti rains down, forming little paper puddles beneath the feet of revelers. In the middle of the celebrations and New Year's kisses, David pauses, reaches into his pocket and pulls out a neatly folded piece of paper. He unfolds the secret note to himself and tightly closes his eyes with an intense focus. *This year will be different*, he promises himself. When he opens his eyes after a few moments, he peers down at his paper, the crowd around him completely oblivious to his inner turmoil.

New Year's Resolutions

1. Get a gym membership

2. Lose 40 pounds

3. Focus on my health

4. Be happy

Seems straightforward enough, right? Here's the problem

though: David's been making the same list for years—for as long as he can remember, actually. Quite frankly, he could've skipped the brainstorming, saved some paper and recycled last year's list. However, there is one difference this time around. This year's weight loss goal has risen to 40 pounds, up from 30 pounds last year. It might not be an identical list, but the underlying themes have remained the same. Get healthy. Get happy. Get lean. Will it be different this time?

David made his list for the first time a few years after graduating from college. While he was in college, he was a successful student-athlete, but like many other college students, he loved to party. It was college, after all. The time eventually came when David had to hang up his jersey, shelve his cleats and join corporate America. Everything that had defined his life changed overnight. Jerseys were swapped with business suits. Out with cleats and headbands, and in with dress shoes and ties. There was no more running and cutting along a grassy field for this guy! Instead, David sat in an office clicking a mouse and typing at his desk. Water breaks were replaced by coffee breaks. David's comparatively stress-free life as a student-athlete was replaced with deadlines, long work hours and traffic.

Stress-free? Well, maybe it *was* stressful being a student-athlete who had to keep performing in the classroom in order to make it onto the field in the first place, but now, compared to his office job, David wishes he could go back to those good ol' days. His only escape from his job these days is Friday and Saturday nights. (Well, okay, if he's totally honest with himself, sometimes it's Wednesday and Thursday nights too.) When David lets loose, he relives old times with friends, the local bars, fast food and a never-ending supply of stories. Sleep? That's what coffee and energy drinks are for! (At least *that* hasn't changed much since college.)

But as the years fly by while sitting in corporate America, David suddenly notices that his waistline is increasing at a much faster rate than his salary. When he was a student-athlete, it was easy to stay in shape. Now David is overweight, doesn't fit his favorite clothes and feels fat. At least he's making good money, though ... Right?

The first time David made his New Year's resolution list, he tried his favorite celebrity's approach that he read about in a magazine. After a few weeks, the results weren't what the magazine promised, and the whole plan fell apart. The next year, it was a fitness guru from a trendy bodybuilding website he stumbled across who 'provided the path to optimal health and wellness'. Like magic, the workout plan came alongside a supplement that would allow him eat anything he wanted and still lose weight. That one failed too. The following year, it was a smiling face on a DVD cover—with matching chiseled abs to boot—who guaranteed David would 'lose that belly fat and shred those abs' in just six minutes a day. That effort lasted just six days – and his stomach looked nothing like the DVD cover. The year after that, he bought a gym membership, hired a nutritionist and even got alongside a personal trainer to jump-start his routine. The year after that... Well, you get the picture.

Year after year, David found himself drifting farther and farther away from his health and wellness goals. He looked at himself in the mirror and wondered how the weight gain had happened so quickly. He swears he never noticed it creep on. It just sort of ... happened. David glanced down at his four resolutions knowing he was very far from being healthy, happy and lean. He was unhealthy, depressed and fat. If things didn't change soon, David would soon be labeled as obese. And that was an even bigger problem.

...

Too many people, irrespective of whether they're fat or thin, regard obesity simply as a cosmetic issue. Society is filled with people who try one diet or drug after another in an attempt to conform to society's accepted standards of beauty—or perhaps more accurately, a Photoshop programmer's standard of beauty. What people fail to realize, though, is that obesity is actually a serious health problem that's not restricted to the mirror.

Look around and you're likely to see obesity everywhere. What was once a rare sight has now evolved into a commonplace occurrence because society has conditioned us into eating more and exercising less. But obesity isn't just a cosmetic thing that affects how you look in a dress; first and foremost it's a serious health problem that has been linked to many chronic diseases, some that ultimately result in death. Consequently, people who are obese are more likely to suffer from the kinds of chronic and degenerative diseases Americans face today.[1,2,3] It's one of the biggest problems our country currently faces, and it generally results from the lifestyle choices that we make every day.[4] The saddest part of these grim realities is that many chronic diseases, along with obesity, are preventable. It all begins with lifestyle.

Your lifestyle is the sum of all the individual choices you make throughout the day. Of course it's what you eat, but it's also how you move, feel, sleep, think, learn and live. All of it counts because every choice matters. Lifestyle is the collective whole of how you live your life.

So there's a reason—several reasons—why David's New Year resolutions have been playing on repeat. He didn't go to bed at night skinny and wake up overweight. For many, it may seem like massive weight gain did happen overnight—you may be nodding your head in agreement as you read this—but that's what happens when someone simply stops paying long-term attention to their health. They wake up one day and wonder what happened. The reality is that there was a process, a series of intermediary steps, that went from lean to overweight and on to obese. Like David, things got out of hand—one lifestyle decision at a time.

David was overweight because he ate processed chemicals posing as food instead of *real* food. He was overweight because he hated his job, lived alone and argued with his girlfriend every day. He was overweight because he didn't have time to work out today… for the last six months. He was overweight because he never got a good night's rest and needed coffee to keep his eyes open. He was overweight because he drank more beer and mixed drinks than he did water. It wasn't just one thing that made him overweight; it was his entire lifestyle.

Every decision David made in the past and each one he makes moving forward will impact his health. Health is not a status to be acquired or a milestone to reach, but rather a relationship between an individual and his external and internal environments. Health is the relationship you have with your body, and David's relationship is struggling because he doesn't give his body what it needs to thrive. David's been neglecting this relationship for a long time. If he doesn't change something soon, his lifestyle choices that have virtually become second-nature could seriously harm—or kill—him.

You've heard the statistics before, but here they one more time for good measure. In 2010, the Center for Disease Control and Prevention reported that 36% of U.S. men and women were obese and another 33% are on their way there, already overweight.[5] That means over 200 million people in the United States are either overweight or obese. To put it lightly, that's frightening. Overall, less than a third of the adult population maintains a healthy weight their entire life. When you look at it that way, it makes sense that so many New Year resolutions look identical. But obesity isn't an aesthetic issue. It's a serious health problem that is quickly impacting not just America's adult population, but also our future generations—and our national economy.

For the first time in two centuries, the current generation of children in America may have shorter life expectancies than their parents, thanks to the prevalence and severity of obesity. Over 30% of America's children and adolescents have joined the obesity ranks, making them more likely to suffer from diseases and complications such as type 2 diabetes, heart disease, kidney failure and cancer at younger and younger ages.[6]

Yep, you read it right. Today, American children actually have a shorter life expectancy than their parents. An Oxford University study found that obesity reduces life expectancy by as much as 10 years. This is similar to the effects that a lifelong smoker might experience.[7] Put simply, obesity is unhealthy. There's no way around it. There's obviously a whole lot more riding on the decision to 'lose a few pounds' than fitting into tight jeans or getting ready for bikini season. It's your health that's on the line.

Why Focus on Fat?

The truth is that we could swap out obesity for any other chronic disease, and lifestyle would still remain the main focus of cause, treatment and prevention. While medical interventions are necessary for clinical-level symptoms and diseases, a healthy lifestyle works alongside these treatment strategies, regardless of severity. So why are we focusing on obesity and weight management as opposed to other chronic conditions like type 2 diabetes or Alzheimer's? The answer has everything to do with measurability and giving the individual the power to assess their own progress.

Ask some people what it is they really want to improve in their lives, and they might answer energy levels, cognitive focus, sexual vitality, sleep quality and overall happiness. While these are essential points to focus on when transforming your life, they're also very subjective and therefore very hard to measure. Obesity, on the other hand, is a unique chronic condition because it provides objective, measureable and quantifiable tracking abilities without the need for expensive and invasive medical procedures. You don't always need inconvenient and sometimes invasive blood work or lab tests to assess your own progress. Just hop on a scale, use a tape measure or feel how your clothes fit differently. The results of lifestyle interventions are visible in the mirror; you don't need an expert to tell you that you're getting leaner.

Take a look at variables like weight, BMI, circumference measurements and body fat percentage. Practically speaking, body fat percentage has been shown to be the most effective in distinguishing between healthy and obese individuals since it has a greater ability to differentiate between lean mass and fat mass when compared to BMI.[8] Studies have also shown that muscle mass is a better predictor for longevity in adults.[9]

For example, an extremely skinny woman with little or no lean mass will record a healthy BMI even though her body fat percentage is at unhealthy low levels, while an extremely fit American football player with significant lean mass could actually measure an obese-level BMI, even though his body fat percentage is at a healthy level. Lean mass is healthy and thus should be accounted for when assessing body composition.

This quantitative information allows you to assess, measure and compare objective data points, providing a quick check-in to see how your health has changed over time without costly and sometimes unwarranted trips to the doctor's office. Of course, *compare* is the operative word in the previous sentence. Data is just data. It's just a number on a piece of paper. If you learn your body fat percentage today then never measure it again, it really doesn't provide a lot of information. You need a feedback loop to know if your lifestyle is helping you get leaner or contributing to weight gain, towards health or towards disease. Weight-related variables provide an objective approach that can work alongside subjective variables like your energy levels, how often you get sick, sleeping quality and overall level of happiness.

Everyone is different and therefore starts in a different place, so the goal is to track your individual progress over time then compare those numbers to watch yourself get healthier. Tracking weight, body fat percentage or BMI is about improvement and analysis over time, not an arbitrary number that society deems as perfection. It's a *process* that takes you from overweight and unhealthy towards leaner and happier. You don't just jump there overnight.

Fat: It Starts and Ends with Lifestyle

The medical world customarily sees obesity as a diagnosis. In other words, obesity does not become a health problem until the *state* of obesity is actually reached. If you go to the doctor and the chart on the wall shows that you're five pounds below the 'obese' threshold, well then, at least you're not obese, right? *Phew. That was a close one.* This logic is often used for cholesterol, blood sugar and many other markers of human health too. It's not until the test reads a particular number that the health alarms sound. But is this really the best way to look at it? You don't suddenly become unhealthy *after* you get labeled as obese. It's actually the other way around. As you become more and more unhealthy, you move closer and closer towards obesity. It's the unhealthy lifestyles that cause the weight gain that eventually leads to obesity. Just like there's no magic bullet for weight-loss solutions, there's no scapegoat for weight problems either. You've got to look at your entire lifestyle.

Which lifestyle choices are the unhealthiest? Which daily decisions are most associated with weight gain and obesity? In a Serbian study involving 3,854 participants, scientists set out to examine the association between obesity and socioeconomic and lifestyle factors. Was it diet? Lack of physical activity and exercise? Or a combination of those plus more? I think you know the answer. The Serbian researchers concluded that nutrition and exercise plans were an important part of the obesity equation. Certainly the entire world knows about these factors, but the study also found a few interesting lifestyle choices associated with obesity, such as lower educational levels, watching television and being single.[10] It goes without saying that diet and exercise play a critical role in obesity, but it turns out that other aspects of your lifestyle play critical roles as well. Obesity is more than the result of a poor diet and lack of exercise. Social, mental and emotional factors should be considered as well.

It takes a very determined mental mindset and level of emotional awareness to resist stuffing our faces when we're confronted by endless temptation and cravings. Up until only recently, we actually needed our food cravings in order to survive. Humans were biologically designed to consume energy—food—when it was available, then store the excess in fat as an energy reserve. This survival mechanism allowed the human species to survive during the frequent times of famine and low food availability during hunter-gatherer time periods. But the days of hunting and gathering have come and gone, replaced instead by our modern world of ultra-convenience. Our evolutionary advantages have become our curse. Physiological mechanisms at the very core of our brains are designed to prevent starvation, amplify reward and reduce stress, yet they all promote food-seeking and consuming behaviors.[11] When our ancestors found food, they ate it. If they didn't have an immediate need for the energy, they stored it on their bodies in the form of fat. But these days we live in stressful modern day environments with access to unlimited calories, triggering all three of these ancient limbic brain mechanisms at once. Succumbing to food cravings is all but inevitable—that's just how we're wired. We constantly fight deep-rooted primal urges to consume anything that is calorically dense and palatable in our path. Being healthy nowadays requires an integrative lifestyle that acknowledges these primal urges, and uses mind-body techniques to develop self-awareness and self-discipline to overcome such cravings. That's why there's so much more to obesity than just eating less and exercising more.

The same holds true for obesity interventions. Researchers in the United Kingdom reviewed publications in order to investigate the overall effectiveness of lifestyle interventions for the treatment of obesity. The researchers focused mostly on diet, physical activity and psychological behavioral strategies. The meta-analysis found that all—yes, all—lifestyle interventions had a modest but significant effect on weight loss.[12] Surprisingly, there was little evidence to indicate that any one intervention was more effective than the others. They all played an important role.

When determining which lifestyle intervention would be most effective and appropriate, what ultimately matters is the individual.

Which of their current lifestyle choices are the unhealthiest? Is it their diet? Start there. Are they completely sedentary? Create a movement strategy. Is he or she chronically depressed? Consider mental and emotional interventions. An effective healthy lifestyle intervention will differ from person to person. Not surprisingly, the United Kingdom study also concluded that the combination of diet, exercise and behavioral lifestyle interventions implemented in conjunction with one another appeared to be most effective for both the prevention and treatment of obesity. In other words, the whole lifestyle mattered. There's no magic bullet solution.

Your Genetic Poker Hand

While our focus up until now has been obesity, it's important to acknowledge that what we're really talking about is overall health. Health is a dynamic process that ebbs and flows with your lifestyle choices. It's an ongoing process and journey, not a final destination. During that journey, we simply use body composition measurements as check-in points to make sure we're steering the right course. We could just blindly follow instructions, but it's the objective data that will look past our personal biases to see if our methods are actually working.

Put simply, unhealthy lifestyle choices lead a person to becoming overweight, and therefore down the path towards obesity. On the other hand, healthy lifestyles lead to getting leaner and healthier. With every lifestyle choice you make, your body either gets healthier or unhealthier, fatter or leaner. It's the *process* of becoming overweight that matters.

But it's not just lifestyle that matters. Your unique make-up, your DNA, the very matter that makes you, is completely different to the next person. You don't get to pick your genes, even though we've all dreamed what we could have been if we'd had the genetic codes of our favorite athletes or celebrities. Sorry to say it, though, but you're 'stuck' with your genes whether you like it or not.

Imagine you're playing poker. Every player in a poker game will have a different starting hand, dealt out to them completely randomly. The hand you start with is not as important as how you play that hand. In life, it's no different. You get given a starting genetic hand. You can't choose what that hand looks like. Once the game of life starts, however, each and every interaction with the environment—what you eat, how you move, who you love, the air you breathe and the thoughts you hold—impact *how* your genes are expressed. This is the central principle of a branch of science called epigenetics, which literally means *above genes*. What this means is that your daily lifestyle choices impact your body on the most basic genetic level. So while genes (or DNA) hold the blueprints for what your body will look like and how it will function from day to day, each and every lifestyle choice will directly impact how these biological instructions are expressed. Your environment controls how your genes behave. In other words, you're in control, not your genes.

Genes that contribute to many forms of cancer, disease and even obesity actually have to be turned *on* by environmental stimuli. Mounting evidence has shown that genetic susceptibility to obesity and type 2 diabetes can be kept under control by a healthy lifestyle or lifestyle modification. Lifestyle rather than DNA determines whether an individual is more likely to develop the disease.[13] So while you don't get to choose your genes, you do get to choose how significantly they impact your life. This is empowering information because lifestyle choices can improve health, regardless of genetic predisposition. And ultimately, that's the goal we're all looking for: continual improvements to health over our entire lifetimes.

Remember: it's not about perfection, it's about progress and consistency. The more consecutive days of healthy living that you can string together, the greater your improvements to health will be. String together a few months, and you'll have feel like a completely different person. Stay focused for a few years and you'll have the foundation you need for lifelong energy and vitality. But it all starts with taking responsibility of your present circumstances. Regardless of your genetic realities at this very moment, if you can agree that things could be worse—and they can be—then you can also agree that they can be improved. This is where healthy lifestyle choices come in. It starts today. It starts now.

When you draw cards in a poker game, you flirt with chance. You never know if you're one card away from the perfect hand or a total bust. Only the poker gods know that. In life, the cards you draw are your lifestyle choices. How you live your life will either make your hand better or worse, moving towards or further away from health.

The only difference between poker and life is that your lifestyle choices are exactly that: *choices*. Life doesn't come down to probability or luck like poker does. It's the way you live your life and every choice counts. Every decision you make either steers you towards or away from health. If health is a goal in your life, then it must be and will always be a long-term investment on your part. It's a lifelong poker game and the health of your genes is at stake. While there may not be a magic pill, this information should serve to empower you. It means you already have all the tools you need to get healthier. Just like poker, you can choose how to play your starting genetic hand. It's an important choice that will determine your perspective on the world and how you live within it. Will you accept your genetic fate, give up and fold? Or will you play the game of life with the hand you've been dealt, and improve it with every passing moment? You may not have drawn a Royal Flush in terms of your genes, but by focusing on a healthy lifestyle you can *earn* yourself a Full House instead of simply giving up and folding.

The 'now what?' moment has set in right about now, and you're waiting for the punch line. You're asking yourself, *What do I do now? Who is right? Who is wrong? I've tried everything. Plenty of times. Each time something a little different, and each time ended with failure.* You're right. There's just too much information out there. How can anyone possibly filter through the massive amounts of health and wellness information available to the public, then create a health plan that will work 100% of the time?

It may be a chaotic world of information out there, but don't let the endless options be your restraint. You will soon learn how to filter through the endless magazines, articles, celebrity testimonials, news reports and your neighbor's miracle stories that find their way into your mental landscape. Your health will be in your own hands. The answer is to live in accordance with the six Healthy Lifestyle Principles.

Creating Your Own Healthy Lifestyle

Health is the very foundation of happiness. Health is the long-term investment that pays dividends in the form of a healthy body composition, or less body fat and more lean muscle. Invariably when you chase health, you gain aesthetics as a byproduct. Your external appearance becomes an expression of your internal health. But how do you get from point A to point B, from where you are now to the healthiest version of yourself? Navigating that path is not always easy. There are plenty of possible roads, highways, detours and dead-ends. But which map is *right?*

Do you want to lose weight by going vegan or vegetarian? Just Google 'vegan for weight loss' and you'll find emotionally-charged documentaries and doctors galore. Want to lose weight following the Paleo diet? Google it and you'll find great testimonials and peer-reviewed research studies aplenty. Want to lose weight doing yoga? Google says that yoga is the best tool for fat loss. Want to lose weight running? Yep, you guessed it: Google tells you that running is the best tool for fat loss too. And is it high-fat, high-protein or high-carb that does the trick for belly fat? All of them apparently. Or none of them, depending on which phrase you search.

The internet is a wonderful thing, but it can be pretty confusing too. A quick online search will confirm any ideology you might be debating. Even the most credible scholars disagree with each another on certain topics. Every successive search will spotlight studies, doctors, personal testimonials and statistics to prove its almighty supremacy over every other health and wellness ideology. Beliefs that fall outside of their ideology will be judged as inferior, and doom all those who follow it to a horrible and painful death. Health and wellness ideologies are just the newest rendition of religious disagreements that often lead to similarly passionate debates.

But just to confuse you further, it's ironic that when you add 'bad' or 'dangers of' to your original online search, you'll often get just as many results with equally compelling doctors, personal testimonials and statistics telling you about the problems associated with these methodologies. *So who's right and who's wrong?*

Here's the first important lesson to learn before turning the next page: no one has the claim to absolute health and wellness truth or complete knowledge. No one. The bottom line is that you must learn to think for yourself. Only then will you claim full control over your health.

The truth is that what is and what's not healthy for any given person totally depends on the individual. We're all different, so we need to understand our own bodies in order to be healthy. Sure, there are great tips and tricks you'll learn along the way from many brilliant teachers who have walked the walk and talked the talk, but without a fundamental understanding of your own body, those tricks and tips will be short lived and temporary quick fixes rather than sustainable lifestyles.

When someone tells you to eat something they believe to be healthy, you need to ask the right questions and evaluate the situation for yourself without mindlessly accepting the health claim as truth (see *Real Food*). When your best friend asks you to try the hottest new workout, you need to understand what the purpose of movement really is and whether the proposed workout adds to or detracts from your personal needs, wants and goals for physical fitness (see *Movement*). When a bet is on the poker table, people play their own hands. Would you let someone else play your poker hand? Of course you wouldn't. That's why you need to understand the six Healthy Lifestyle Principles. Armed with these principles, *you* will be the master and commander of your own ship, no one else. The best lifestyle strategy is to place your faith in yourself. Your body will never lie.

Healthy Lifestyle Principles focus on fundamental human needs. They're what you *need* for health, not what you might want, like or find convenient. Technically, these principles should be self-evident and obvious, but unfortunately they're not. Collectively, we've actually forgotten how to live optimally. By focusing intently on the complexities of modern life, we've let our basic human functions fall by the wayside. We can build complex mobile applications for smartphones, talk about the latest and greatest features of the newest television technology, and even know what top best matches those heels, but when it comes to health, we don't know anything. We've lost the inherent connection to our own bodies—at the expense of our health. We don't know how to identify real food that is actually healthy. We sit at a desk all day, even though evolution dictates we should be exploring the outdoors and moving. We live in small rooms, interact with people over social media rather than face-to-face, and connect with nature is through a National Geographic TV show. It's time to revisit and learn the fundamental qualities that characterize the life of every healthy person on this planet.

Healthy Lifestyle Principles provide a general framework for what healthy lifestyles should look like, much like a building's blueprints. A blueprint is a plan of action. When constructing a modern architectural marvel such as a skyscraper, blueprints provide the measurements, calculations and layout to ensure that the building is constructed with a strong foundation. Blueprints are the specific directions needed to create a building's most important structures. Failing to comply with blueprints will lead to major costs and more work to correct, if the job gets done at all. The six Healthy Lifestyle Principles are your guide to getting healthier, happier and leaner, regardless of your starting point. Without fail, you will find that the healthiest people around you and around the world live their lives in accordance with these six Healthy Lifestyle Principles (HLP).

HLP #1: Real Food
Forget fad diets; focus on lifestyle. Paleo? Vegan? It really doesn't

matter. When you look at the bigger picture of Real Food, you'll discover why putting nature's own produce into your body is so much better than processed convenience quasi-food. In this chapter you'll learn how to identify *real* food, something that's quickly becoming a lost art. When you can confidently determine whether the plate on your table add to or detracts from to your health, you will gain the key to improving your health.

HLP #2: Movement

We've all been told how important it is to exercise every day, but we've also all come up with a range of reasons why we don't do it. Daily movement isn't just for exercise benefits, though. It's actually the key to well-rounded health. Humans were born to move, and the increased flexibility and circulation that comes with daily movement is essential for optimal health. But we're all different. Choose a program and mode of movement that works for you, don't just do what everyone else does and assume you'll enjoy the same results. In the end, it's just about getting up and doing something every single day. Just move.

HLP #3: Rest & Relaxation

Close your eyes and picture your car. You drive it every single day. You take corners too quickly and brake heavily. You forget to keep the engine topped up with oil. You scrape along the side of the garage every now and again. But the busyness of life means you never have the time to take it into a mechanic for a service, oil change or repairs. What's going to happen? That's right; it's going to break down. Your body's just the same. Treat it badly, and it'll respond badly. Put it under too much stress, and you'll discover an array of issues you never knew existed. But implement restorative strategies, and your body will have the opportunity to combat the detrimental effects of stress, thus rejuvenating and reviving itself. In this chapter you'll learn how to create a lifestyle that combines good levels of work and rest so you won't get more fatigued or stressed than you need to be—because life is about having fun alongside your responsibilities and commitments.

HLP #4: Lifelong Learning

Mark Twain once said, "Don't let schooling interfere with education." We often forget the power of learning when Google is so accessible. But online 'education' at our fingertips is not enough. To achieve a life of health, you need to stay involved in your own lifelong educational journeys. Education doesn't end with the presentation of a framed piece of expensive paper; learning is the tool that enhances every aspect of life. Healthy living is a process, not a goal. It requires extensive use of your brainpower. Use it or lose it.

HLP #5: Community

Humans evolved as social creatures. In fact, social connection is fundamental to the human race's evolutionary success. In every level of organization, from atomic to cellular to societal, cooperative social relationships create prosperity. Communities provide structure, purpose and camaraderie, and can actually enhance the lives of the entire group. It's time to take down your walls, let go of fear, turn off your computer and cellphone, and embrace one of the fundamental human needs: face-to-face social connection.

HLP #6: Love

'Love' is one of the most ambiguous terms in the English language: you can love your soul mate, your cat, your car and a stunning view all at the same time, yet the level of love you experience is different for all of them. But love, in relation to Healthy Lifestyle Principles, is the glue that holds a healthy lifestyle together, and it exists all around you all the time. Embrace the present moment. Learn how to love yourself, your journey, your surroundings and your emotions—all of them—and every aspect of your life will be transformed.

...

While these six Healthy Lifestyle Principles are integral to a lifelong healthy lifestyle, every single person will apply them to their own lives differently. We all come from a melting pot of genetic combinations, ethnic blending and differently-knit social cultures and communities. One person might choose to eat Paleo while another might become strictly vegan. We all have different fitness goals. Someone who's looking for improved flexibility might choose yoga over traditional strength training, especially if they're also trying to incorporate more meditative and relaxation strategies into their life (see *Rest and Relaxation*).

We're also physiologically different. From differences in organ sizes and lengths, to microbial populations and species in our guts, right through to hormones, enzymes and biochemical individuality; even a person's physical structure and posture can tell their unique life story, with every lifestyle decision they've made culminating into the single moment of the present.

How can a single diet, a single workout, or any single lifestyle choice apply to everyone universally? Well, it can't. The possibilities and options for healthy lifestyles are endless. As long as those lifestyle choices align with the six fundamental Healthy Living Principles, then it really doesn't matter what you do as long as it focused on *you*. Did your meal make you sick? Bloated? Gassy? *Time to investigate further.* Did that workout make your shoulder hurt? Pull a hamstring? *Time to investigate further.* Constant questioning and experimentation will help you reconnect with your body. It's a process of trial and error that teaches you something with every passing moment (see *Lifelong Learning*). It's not about getting it right every time, it's about process and progress.

It's never too late to choose a life of health, vitality and energy. It's never too late to thrive. When you begin to live your life in alignment with the six Healthy Living Principles, your body will flourish again. Indeed, studies show that as you age, healthy lifestyles become more important for longevity.[14,15] If you can accept with full confidence that your current situation could be worse—which it could be—then it logically follows that your current situation could also be better.

Health is a process. A process which starts with a choice. Always remember that your degree of success is about progress, not perfection. With every lifestyle choice you make, your situation either becomes better or worse. But rest assured that your body *always* chooses health if you put it in a healthy environment. Survival is the only thing your body knows how to do.

Your mind may understand it has several purposes (eat, drink, work, relax, party, dance), but your body only knows one: survival. When you sleep, your body replenishes itself. When you cut yourself, you scab up, which is your body's way to repair. If you eat something that disagrees with your system, your body will expel it. When it's given the opportunity to do its job properly, your body really knows what it's doing. It's time, then, that you get on the same page and help support the natural healing processes that your body has initiated since you were born. Your body's innate wisdom is greater than anyone has led you to believe. Learn to trust it. It's time to center your life on the six Healthy Lifestyle Principles. Healthy living is your birthright.

A Million Ways to Live

If there's only one thing you take from this book, know that being healthy—or rather the *process* of becoming *healthier*—is going to look different for each and every person. Depending on where you live, who and what you interact with on a daily basis, and the many other intricate facets of life, each individual is faced with diverse experiences in a wide variety of environments. If you travel around the world you'll see these principles being implemented in so many different ways. Different cultures, local environments and unique tastes all play their role in expressing the principles of healthy living. There's no one right answer, though. There's no one-size-fits-all solution. We *need* a million ways to live because of the important link between diversity and health.

Within every macro and micro level system, the concept of diversity is found at the very core of the health of that system. The most stable ecosystems are the ones with the widest variety of plant and animal species. In the event of an environmental disaster, the ecosystem that is the most diverse will always have the greatest chance of survival. Diversity of thought encourages new ideas to be imagined that can be beneficial to a society—even the world. Even your personal financial investments need diversity to flourish; that's why mutual funds are often considered the safest stock market investments. We need diversity in every aspect of our lives. If everyone lived the same way, the human race wouldn't live for long.

When it comes to lifestyles, all humans have a basic need to express themselves, to show others who they are, what they stand for, how they're different. This is what makes them special, unique and irreplaceable. People choose to express themselves differently based on their backgrounds, personalities, culture and attitude. Individuality and diversity is important because new ideas stem from differing viewpoints. Multiple solutions need to be considered for single problems in order to solve them in the most efficient ways.

Individuality makes life interesting and exciting. Without it, the world would be a very stagnant and, quite frankly, boring place. Therefore, create a lifestyle that's best suited for you, that will excite you when you when you wake up in the morning. We're all trying to achieve the same goal of health, but everyone carries with them a lifetime of stories and experiences that finely chisel the finishing touches on their respective individualities. We may have the same blueprints for a healthy life, but it is our inner authentic self that puts the finishing touches on our home. There are no universal answers that work all the time for every tough situation. There's no right way to live. There has never been and never will be. There are a million ways to live.

The world is your oyster, but you have to take those first daring steps if you want to succeed. If you want a future defined by health tomorrow, the bottom line is that you have to change your lifestyle today. You can't expect different outcomes when you keep doing the same things day after day. Remember, like a poker hand, we all have different starting points. But once you take responsibility for your own health, you get to dictate what happens next. You get to play your own poker hand.

You have the power to make things better. Strive for progress, not perfection. Don't get down on yourself if you mess up here and there. It's normal. It's human. It's life.

Just stay focused on the six Healthy Lifestyle Principles and move forward. Progress breeds momentum, which in turn breeds success. Identify the principle that you need most help with or want to pay more attention to, then improve this aspect of your life one habit at a time. It's an enjoyable educational process that promises to make every moment of the rest of your life sweeter and more fulfilling. The greatest wealth is health. And it's a fruit all of us have the power to taste.

It's time for your Lifestyle Transformation.

Real Food

"To eat is a necessity, but to eat intelligently is an art." – La Rochefoucauld

"Tell me what you eat, and I will tell you who you are." – Jean Brillat-Savarin

Welcome to day one of David's health and wellness transformation. David is motivated, inspired, and ready to kick-start his healthy lifestyle. Like most people, he decides to tackle his diet first, since 'a healthy lifestyle starts in the kitchen,' or at least that's what he's heard. *This is going to be a piece of cake*, he says to himself as he parks his car and heads towards the supermarket entrance. *How hard can it be to shop for healthy food?*

As he grabs a shopping cart and casually pushes it through the sliding glass doors, he hums confidently and calmly to himself, a self-assured smile playing at his lips. Suddenly, David stops in the center of the fruit and vegetable section. He's unexpectedly confronted by the enormity of this unfamiliar situation. He looks left then right then left again. Reality sets in. Inside the gigantic, over-lit and quite frankly intimidating supermarket are endless aisles filled with thousands upon thousands of products. David shakes his head as he struggles to think straight amidst the endless chattering of beeps from cashiers scanning food products. Anguish suddenly overwhelms him. The truth is, David can't remember the last time he bought groceries for himself, let alone *healthy* groceries. And now, with this seemingly infinite array of options, he has absolutely no idea where to start. Which things are healthy?

Where should he look first? How should he compare options? *Uh oh, maybe this won't be as easy as I thought*, he sighs.

As David trudges aimlessly along the aisles and gazes left to right then left again, searching for direction, the weight of the world gradually drops from his shoulders as he breathes a huge sigh of relief. *Actually, grocery shopping really isn't that difficult after all.* Even though David has no idea where to start, all is good in the world because the products lining the supermarket shelves all have colorful labels on them that proudly proclaim their health benefits. 99% fat free! Reduces cholesterol! Less sugar than another similar product! *Huh, who would have thought eating healthy was this easy?! I should have done this whole 'healthy eating' thing ages ago!*

So David confidently strolls down the supermarket aisles, stopping when bright colors and buzzwords catch his attention. By the time he reaches the checkout line, he gives himself a mental high-five and unloads his cart onto the conveyor belt one item at a time. First up, a six-pack of diet soda (*zero calories? Count me in!*). Next, some margarine (*the package said 'heart healthy' and 'cholesterol-free' so that's got to be good, right?*). A box of berry-flavored cereal bars (*high in fiber and low in calories—that sounds about right!*). A pint of organic ice cream (*I heard somewhere that organic is healthier*). A brand name green smoothie drink (*the bottle said it would make me into a green machine!*). David drives home feeling accomplished.

David wonders why so many people struggle with the whole 'eating healthy' thing when the supermarket makes it so easy to find healthy food. *All you've got to do is read the labels!*

...

Despite David's triumphant feeling of accomplishment, his trip to the grocery store actually resulted in purchases that weren't so healthy after all. For example, margarine actually contains high amounts of partially hydrogenated oils, the consumption of which has been proven to contribute to metabolic disorders and chronic diseases like cancer and coronary heart disease.[1,2,3,4] Commonly known as trans-fats, these harmful industrially-manufactured products have created a stigma around natural trans-fats, which are found in natural grass-fed dairy and meat products and have been shown to prevent cancer and be beneficial for all-round health.[5,6,7,8]

David's other food choices aren't much better. Some artificial sweeteners used in diet soda have been clinically linked to cognitive dysfunction, obesity and endocrine system dysfunction.[9,10,11,12,13,14] On top of that, diet sodas just don't work well as a health and weight loss strategy.[15] Cereal bars have high amounts of sugar and can hinder the body's digestive functions. Whether it's organic or not, ice cream is just not the healthiest choice for a person attempting to lose weight and get healthy. That green smoothie might promise a lot of things, but it's packed with sugar, which directly contributes to weight gain and inflammation.

And yet, David left the grocery store certain he had bought great food options for his new healthy lifestyle goals. The truth is that many of us face these same predicaments every time we enter the supermarket. People everywhere unintentionally make dietary choices that prevent them from reaching their true health potential. It's easy to blame the food companies that manufacture these products, but that would be too easy.

Healthy eating has become so confusing you'd think a Master's degree is required to understand the topic. Some people rely on colorful labels and marketing slogans to tell them the nutritional value of what they're eating. *The box said it was heart-healthy.*

Others need their smartphone apps for the green light on their food choices. Others consult nutritionists, doctors or dieticians for advice on what they should eat and when; they'd feel lost unless an expert blessed each morsel that entered their mouths. When did eating become such a complicated process? Or have we become so disconnected from food that we literally don't know how to eat and live healthy anymore?

It's probably not too hard to believe that humans, like any other living organism, have been successfully eating for hundreds of thousands of years. By utilizing natural instincts, time-tested traditions and geo-specific food cultures, human populations have prospered all around the world. It's only been in the last hundred years or so that we've complicated the eating process to a point where we don't know what real food looks like anymore. Instead we opt for food-like substitutes claiming to be nutritionally equivalent or superior to Mother Nature's originals. Marketing and bioengineering have replaced common sense and generations of proven methodologies. As a result, both individual and environmental health has suffered.

Becoming healthier isn't just about eating the right things; it actually means reconnecting with the entire food experience, from start to finish, farm to plate, and soil to shelf. It's about understanding where food comes from and, more importantly, what constitutes real food. Only then can an individual quickly and effectively identify whether the foods they're eating will heal or harm their bodies. Turn your backs on marketing executives and their flashy labels designed to influence your food buying decision. If you want to walk through the sliding glass door of a supermarket and know you can make healthy selections, you have to focus on finding real food.

Just Eat Real Food

It's time to get a little scientific. Your body is made up of an estimated 37 trillion cells.[16] That's 37,200,000,000,000 cells, just so you can see how large that number truly is. Every day, tens (or hundreds, depending on who you ask) of billions of these cells die due to apoptosis, or programmed cell death.[17] Just as quickly as your cells die, however, others are created to fill the gaps. Your body is literally a manufacturer of its own cells.

But where do we get the raw materials for such an important manufacturing project?

You've probably heard this famous—and overused—quote that encourages healthy eating habits: *you are what you eat.* Unfortunately the more you hear and see it, the less of an impact it has. But this saying is much more than just an Internet meme shared on social networks. On a fundamental level, you actually *are* what you eat. Just like houses are built from planks of wood that no longer look like trees, the food you eat provides the raw material—in the form of digested nutrients—to build new cells, even though you don't actually look like the food you consume. We constantly replace and reshape our biochemical physiology with the foods we choose to eat, and just like any construction project, the quality of raw material matters.

While many homes may look similar on the outside, it's the foundation of the home that determines how well it holds up against environmental conditions, seasonal changes, and the ordinary wear and tear of the people living inside. You can live in a house with a weak or unstable foundation. You can even decorate it and make it look nice for houseguests. But pretty blinds and matching shades won't do much against an earthquake or hurricane if the frame of the home is compromised. If the foundation of the home is shaky, it won't withstand the test of time or unexpected natural disasters. This is how the human body works too. The structure and foundation of the inside is more important than the aesthetics outside.

The quality of the food we eat determines how strong our foundation is and how well it can weather life's storms. How quickly do you recover from the common cold? How often do you get sick? How long does it take to recover from a workout? These are seemingly small and insubstantial questions, yet they're intimately connected with the foundation of your body. The higher the quality of food you ingest, the stronger your body's foundation will be. While your body can function on a poor diet, it's remarkably more resilient and adaptive to external changes, such as a pesky cold, a nagging flu or an intense workout, when it's built on a dietary foundation of real food.

Instead of a specific definition, it's better to outline the qualities and characteristics of real food so you can determine the 'realness' of the food on your plate. For starters, real food spoils. The general rule of thumb is that if it has a long shelf life, it will shorten yours. Real food doesn't need colorful packaging, logos or marketing slogans. When a product tries hard to convince you of its health benefits, it probably has a large marketing budget behind it. The inherent healthiness of real food speaks for itself; it doesn't require additions or fortifications. Real food is best grown organically—for a variety of reasons, not just your personal health (see *Truly Sustainable Living*)—and purchased from local sources. Real food doesn't need to be cooked to be edible; it can be eaten raw. Real food is whole, unprocessed and as close to its natural state as possible.

It sounds simple and straightforward, but if it was easy, everyone would be eating real food and many of our current health woes wouldn't exist. When you walk into a grocery store, it can be overwhelming and confusing. Just ask David. Supermarket shelves are stacked with edible food-like products that claim and assert their nutritional prowess, and have colorful slogans and mascots to boot. Many large food companies have made the process of finding real, whole and natural food difficult. Since food production processes are hidden behind corporate veils of secrecy, most consumers are simply unaware of the products they are purchasing. They do not read—or understand—the fine print on the nutrition label and are left to rely on a few buzzwords printed on the product's box.

The modern world has severed the most important relationship we have with the external environment: the relationship between our bodies and our food. While every other animal on earth relies on instinct and intuition to guide its food consumption decisions, humans rely on nutritional labels to tell them whether a food is healthy or not. As you begin to eat a diet of real food, you will find that your natural instincts will develop and your intuition will improve, but that takes a little time and experience. You can't expect to rekindle a relationship with food overnight when you've ignored it for 10, 20 or even 30 years. It starts with a process of real food reeducation.

Before your dietary decisions become as second nature as brushing your teeth, start the food reeducation and reconnection process with three little questions. Every time you sit down to eat, look at the plate in front of you and ask yourself: *What is it? Where did it come from? How was it prepared?* At the root of a healthy lifestyle is healthy eating. At the root of healthy eating you will always find real food. The first step in identifying real food—and building your body's foundation with the strongest of raw materials—starts with the first question. *What is it?*

Count Chemicals, Not Calories

You already know what real food looks like. The basic food groups of **fruits, vegetables, meat, dairy, nuts, grains and legumes** all come to mind. Each of these food groups carries its own healthful qualities and plays different roles in building a solid foundation for the human body. This is where you'll find the raw materials you need to build your 'home'. If you use the right ones you'll create and maintain a sturdy foundation that won't easily break down.

When you ask yourself *what is it?* and you answer with one of the food groups listed above, then you're off to a good start. But that's not what makes this question difficult to understand and practice. What you have to watch out for is what's being *added* to your food. This can make all the difference and turn a healthy food selection into an unhealthy one.

Trusting the Package

When you pick up a food item from a shelf, ignore the front of the package and go straight to the nutrition label. This is where you'll find which and how many chemicals, additives or preservatives have been used in the processing of the food. These extras are what make all the difference. Let's use nuts as an example. While each nut variant has inherently different health benefits, as a whole nuts contain healthy fats. Eating a handful of nuts a day will naturally lower cholesterol and provide your body with heart-healthy nutrients. They are so vital to health that you'd probably never catch a Seventh Day Adventist from Loma Linda without them. A 34,000-person study was conducted to identify which healthy habits and lifestyles had the greatest impact on the longevity on this subculture of people who are widely recognized as some of the healthiest people on the planet. Researchers found that for Loma

Linda's Seventh Day Adventists, maintaining a healthy diet, abstaining from smoking and participating in regular exercise were important, but their most important healthy habit was eating nuts, which added 2.74 more years onto their lives.[18]

But it's easy to take real food like nuts and turn it into junk food with just a few small additions. We reach for chocolate covered or honey-roasted varieties because they taste sweeter. *Hey, they're still nuts right?* Or we get nuts that have been flavored, salted or cooked in partially hydrogenated oils that cause heart disease.[19] While some of these mistakes are obvious to the naked eye—as much as we'd like to ignore the thick chocolate coating on the almond—many of the additions require a quick browse of the nutrition label. Does this chemical belong in here? Was this oil ideal for cooking? And what the heck does 'natural flavor' mean? Aren't I eating an almond? Shouldn't the flavor of the almond be natural enough?

Adding Sauce & Condiments

A chicken salad with varieties of vegetables sounds like a healthy option for lunch. Until it's swimming in pools of ranch dressing or teriyaki sauce, that is. Sauces, dressings and condiments tantalize the taste buds, but can turn healthy meals into dishes that would be better served at dessert when you realize how much sugar is on the plate. Think back to the last time you ate sushi. Rather than focusing on the quality and taste of the fish, popular rolls on the menus of many sushi bars are lathered in sweet sauces and rich mayo. We've trained our taste buds to expect explosions of flavors with every bite, leaving us numb to the natural flavors of real food. Even the natural sweetness of fruit seems bland compared to the processed faux-foods we consume daily. Real food may seem bland at first, but that's only because our brains are accustomed to—or addicted to—the flavor rushes that make them more like candy than nourishing meals.

Whether they're used as an additive or condiment, these extras have significant impacts on our bodies. Excessive amounts of refined sugars—like those found in chocolate coverings, glazing sauces and dressings—can quickly add up to extra pounds and lead down the path towards chronic disease.[20] As a chief component of most processed foods, sugar has become the most abused drug in the world. It's an addiction that is as hard to kick as it is unhealthy. Then there are 'natural flavors' like MSG that create insatiable cravings, leading to over-consumption behaviors that have been linked to a host of other health issues, including obesity.[21,22,23] Rather than a feeling of satiety after a snack or meal, these chemicals make you reach for more, blunting the intimate connection between gut and brain.[24,25]

Our connection with our food is already damaged, if not completely broken. Food-like products that flood the market with artificial ingredients override your body's natural communication pathways with chemicals that are designed to be addictive rather than nourishing. These foods are manufactured with profit-maximization in mind, not consumer-health.

The consumption of real food breaks the addiction and allows your body's natural intelligence to reclaim authority over dietary decisions. Real food that is whole, fresh, natural, unrefined and unprocessed will build long-term health. The best options have one-word ingredient lists, like 'kale', 'walnuts,' 'blueberries' or 'salmon.' Your body really is a temple, and to keep that temple strong and resilient you've got to choose the right foods.

...

By asking *what is it?* you'll become more aware of your food choices and greatly enhance your ability to control dietary diversity. This is an important concept because eating wide varieties of foods provides your body with the different combinations of nutrients your body needs to function and thrive. Eating meat provides ample amounts of protein and important nutrients like iron, zinc and selenium, plus it plays an important role in muscle, skin and joint health.[26,27] Fruits and vegetables provide important vitamins and minerals, as well as powerful antioxidants that can help fend off chronic diseases like cancer and heart disease.[28] Nuts provide an excellent energy-dense food choice delivering hypocholesterolemic, cardioprotective, anti-inflammatory and antidiabetic benefits, to name just a few of their powerful qualities.[29] There's no magic bullet, no one food type that will change your life, no single food that holds the secret to health and longevity. Dietary diversity is what matters: lots of different single-ingredient real foods eaten alone or in delicious, fresh concoctions created right in your own kitchen. For every color, shape and kind of fruit, vegetable and animal product, there is a unique health benefit that will contribute to your body's foundation of health. Eat them all.

Look at your body as an ever-expanding database of information. Every time you eat from a wide variety of food sources, your body receives different information from your food, including vitamins, minerals and nutrients. We still don't know and fully understand the complex and intimate relationship between our bodies and the food we eat, but it's safe to say it is much more profound than we can currently validate with present technology. If the only factors that defined real food were nutrients, nutritional supplements and fortified foods would be comparable to real food. Scientific studies, however, confirm that is not the case. The vitamins and minerals in real food are simply more bioavailable and absorbable when consumed whole than when taken as a supplement.[30]

We don't know what other information our body's database is receiving when we eat from diverse food sources. What science has proven so far is that the diversity of your dietary choices contributes to your body's nutrient status,[31,32] resilience to disease,[33] and longevity.[34] Aside from physiological benefits, science is also beginning to show that dietary diversity impacts you on psychological levels as well. Generally speaking, the more diverse your diet, the less likely you are to have food cravings. This is an important consideration since all too often it is not our knowledge of healthy food choices that prevents healthy eating habits, but rather cravings for unhealthy foods that keep us coming back for more unhealthy food options.[35] While there is certainly more to food cravings than dietary diversity (see *Love*), a monotonous diet is an easy variable you can control to help establish and strengthen healthy eating behaviors.

There are hundreds (if not thousands) of edible fruits and vegetables on the market. Most people only eat a small spectrum of what is available to them. How many different foods do you eat? Is it less than 10? For most people, it is. Begin the process of diverse and healthy eating by simply asking *what is it?*—every time you take a bite.

Follow the Dirt

Raise your hand if eating is sometimes seen as a bit of an inconvenience. Eating has almost become a necessary evil, something we need to do as quickly as possible so we can appease those inconsiderate stomach growlings then continue on with our busy schedules. Convenience trumps quality when the busyness of life dictates how much time we have available to eat. Is it any wonder, then, why food quality has deteriorated over time? Ask and you shall receive.

The market has responded to our demands of convenience and speed with droves of quick and easy mealtime fixes that let us continue with our busy day—at the expense of our long-term health. We've simply stopped caring. But food is more complex than calories and macronutrient ratios. Food tells a story and the deeper you go and the more you listen, the better off you will be. That's why the second question you must ask when determining the health of your food is *where did it come from?*

When you walk into a grocery store and see neatly packaged food items stacked floor to ceiling, it's easy to forget that your food came from somewhere else first. There isn't a garden or ranch behind the grocery store that supplies the building with food. Instead, food travels from far and wide—locally, nationally and internationally—to reach supermarket shelves, in the process revealing information like the geographical place of origin, the farming method used to grow your food, and even the living conditions of the animal whose meat you are about to consume. All of these factors impact the quality of the food you eat, so it's in your best interest to play food detective and follow the dirt.

Fruits and vegetables are often the first and most attractive choices for seeking health-promoting foods, and rightfully so. When you eat seven or more servings of fruits and vegetables a day, you reduce the risk of death by cancer and heart disease by a whopping 25% and 31% respectively.[36] But to take advantage of and maximize the nutritional benefits of fruits and vegetables, you have to consider how long it has been since these foods were harvested. Fresh food is healthier food. As soon as fruits and vegetables are harvested from their tree, vine or plant, they begin to lose moisture, nutrients begin to degrade and the likelihood of bacterial spoilage increases.[37] As food loses its freshness, its nutritional value decreases. That's why freshly-picked fruits and vegetables will always be the best source of quality vitamins and minerals.

But what happens when you don't have access to freshly picked fruits and vegetables? Modern systems of food distribution transport foods from all over the country—and the world—in order to provide convenience, year-round availability and diversity. When you consider that fruits and vegetables spend days in transit, inventory and finally in the compartments of your refrigerator, this adds up to roughly five to 15 days between harvest and consumption.[35] This is why frozen fruits and vegetables can sometimes be the more practical and nutritious approach for you if you don't have access to fresh produce from local farmer's markets or home gardens.[38,39] Frozen fruits and vegetables have been preserved at their nutritional peak, and their frozen state allows them to retain their nutritional potency,[40,41] not to mention their convenience.

...

When you play food detective and follow the dirt, the trail will eventually lead you to 'organic' farming, an agricultural practice that focuses on growing the healthiest and most nutritious foods from the healthiest and most nutritious soils.[42] Organic eating is a pretty trendy international food trend, so it's important to make sure you know the ins and out of it before naively jumping on the organic bandwagon. The health benefits associated with organic food are directly related to the soil from which it was grown. With a deep understanding of the biological processes involved in organic farming, farmers preserve and improve the productive capacity of soil over time, which means healthier food for you, both now and into the future (see *Truly Sustainable Living*).[43] Putting healthy food on your plate is important, but so too is ensuring that healthy food will be available for generations to come. This is why supporting organic agricultural practices is worth the price difference; you're investing in healthy and fertile soils that will continue to produce food for your children, and their children, and their children.

So what makes organic food better than other fresh whole foods? Organic crops are grown in soil that has higher levels of minerals, phytonutrients, antioxidants and vitamins.[44] Grass-fed livestock raised solely on pasture and hay are healthier for human consumption than their grain-fed counterparts.[45,46] Eggs from free-range chickens allowed to forage outside are more nutrient-dense and healthier than their conventional counterpart.[47] Healthy soil and healthy animals create healthy food, which in turn builds a healthy human body. It's a simple equation to remember when deciding whether to stick with a conventional diet or go organic.

But it's what organic practices avoid that make them superior foods for your health. Let's compare conventional and organic farming for just a second. Conventional farming commonly uses pesticides to maximize crop yields by protecting plants from pests and weeds. While it might be an economically beneficial practice, whether or not pesticides impact human health has been a hotly debated topic for dozens of years.

Pesticides were commercially introduced with maximum productivity and efficiency in mind, not human health. They only offer short-term economic solutions to problems that are inherent to the underlying farming system. Simply put, conventional farming methods that rely on chemicals to boost crop yields are in fact more prone to diseases, weeds and pests that make pesticides an attractive option to begin with. Organic farms, on the other hand, rely on natural systems of control to keep them disease- and pest-free but produce a healthier and higher quality of output. Organic farming requires more farming know-how, not chemical intervention.

Recently, Pesticide Action Network North America (PANNA), an organization working to replace hazardous pesticides with ecologically-sound and socially-just alternatives, examined more than 200 peer-reviewed studies in order to address the true severity of pesticide use and the health consequences they pose for children's health. What they found wasn't pretty. The report, titled *A Generation in Jeopardy*, outlines the breadth and depth of the unfavorable health consequences associated with pesticide exposure, which included evidence for childhood cognitive dysfunction, cancer, asthma, diabetes and obesity.[48] The report found that even small amounts of pesticide exposure during pregnancy or early childhood could have significant health repercussions.

That's undoubtedly a serious health issue, not just for our generation but for ones to come. But despite the reports and the risk, conventional farming continues to gamble with the health of future generations without fully understanding how these chemicals impact human life. Fortunately, emerging science and evidence continues to show the long-term impacts of pesticide exposure that simply have not been available in the past. These findings should serve as powerful evidence for future change to an archaic food system.

Yet another concern is how various pesticides impact human health synergistically. When studies are done on a single pesticide, the aim is to find how it impacts the human body. The issue, though, is that there are often multiple pesticides used within one farming operation, but science simply does not know what happens when these pesticides interact with each other and how they affect the human body. Cross-contamination and pesticide mixture is virtually guaranteed by the time a consumer accesses foods sprayed with pesticides, yet no one really knows just how dangerous the chemical combo actually is.

The long-term ramifications of cross pesticide mixture and contamination need to be extensively researched and considered, but they're often swept aside in favor of short-term economic productivity and big dollars. However, the information that has been gathered so far in environmental studies comes to the conclusion that pesticides are more toxic when combined.[49] And if that's the case, the impact combined toxins have on humans can be assumed to be just as toxic. When your health—and the health of future generations is on the line—it's better to be safe than sorry. Go organic.

...

Taking center stage in local, state and even national political forums is the growing debate of Genetically Modified Foods (GMO). In the last half century, GMO technology has been developed and used in an attempt to increase crop yield, improve drought resistance, enhance nutrient-density or variation, and withstand resistance to herbicide. Despite these improvements in agricultural efficiency and productivity, increasing numbers of medical and health professionals are encouraging their patients and clients to steer clear of GMOs and keep their diet focused predominantly on organic foods. While the reasons to avoid GMOs go much further than simply improving personal health and wellbeing—in particular their environmental and economic impacts (see *Truly Sustainable Living)*—in this section we focus on how GMO consumption is unsafe for human consumption.

Humans have co-evolved with their natural foods for hundreds of thousands of years. It has only been in the last few years that drastic and fundamental changes have been made to the human diet. GMO technology represents the most drastic and fundamental of all the agricultural changes and what we don't understand could impact our long-term personal and environmental health. We must proceed carefully and cautiously with powerful food technology and pay special attention to warning signs that GMO could very realistically cause long-term health ramifications.

The fact of the matter is that there aren't very many studies about the effects GMOs have on humans. What we do know, though, is that GMO crops have been harmful to other animals. One study found that feeding pigs GMO corn and soy resulted in significant gastric and uterine differences, in particular severe stomach inflammation, compared to their non-GMO counterparts.[50] Even though this long-term study was done on pigs, it's important to understand that human and pig digestive systems are very similar; that's why pig fetuses are chosen for dissections in many high school biology classes. A pig's digestive system includes the same organs with the same functions as humans. In another study, the DNA from GMO potatoes was spliced with a snowdrop plant, which resulted in a variant that was poisonous to mammals and damaged vital organs and immune function.[51]

While studies on animals are not directly transferable to humans, the results should raise eyebrows, warning flags and the attention of the public. One of the only significant long-term and independent studies that address the effects of GMO products on humans found that genetically altered foods caused serious and significant organ damage and tumors.[52] Unfortunately, this study received enormous amounts of backlash from the wider scientific community because the testing methods did not conform to internationally-accepted testing protocols, despite the lead researcher's assurance that he used the same processes that are followed in short-term studies that give approval to GMO products to hit the market.

Because there has been so little research undertaken in this area, humans are arguably unassuming guinea pigs in a long-term and ongoing experiment on GMO consumption. We involuntarily participate simply by passively consuming the enormous variety of GMO products already overcrowding our supermarket shelves. We don't know how the altered genes of the foods we eat will impact our physiology in the long-term or how it will impact us on the most fundamental of levels: our genes. Emerging research is beginning to show that plant genes from food have the ability to influence the ongoing expression of genes in mammals after they're ingested.[53] In other words, you should be asking yourself, *how will these genetically modified genes impact my genetic expression, my very being, when they were designed with economic and productivity interests in mind and not potential ramifications on human health?* That's the million-dollar question. Only time and extensive research will tell. Until then, choose organic.

When it comes to playing food detective, following the dirt is very much like going down Alice's rabbit hole. The more questions you ask and the more you dig, the more information you find, which in turn increases the amount of responsibility you have when making food choices. Sometimes you may not like what you learn, but this is the knowledge you will need when you're serious about improving your health. When you consistently ask *where did it come from?* you realize there is much more to food than just picking the right food group. It is, in fact, a story. You begin to hear a narrative of sorts that continually ends with the same punch line: eat local and organic. These concepts are more than just buzz words; they can impact the health of your food, your environment and your body.

Food Prep Matters

You look down at your plate and see a juicy steak, cooked to perfection. You know it came from a local rancher, grazed on grass its entire life, and was slaughtered humanely. Only one question remains before you enjoy your meal. *How was it prepared?*

If you don't think this question is important, just ask one of the estimated 48 million people who get sick from the food they eat.[54] They'll tell you that food preparation is important. Nearly half of all the food disease outbreaks that occur in the United States comes from restaurants or delis where business owners prioritize profits over health.[55] Clearly, food preparation matters when it comes to choosing healthy food.

Sometimes, foods are best eaten uncooked. Milk is one of those foods. When milk is pasteurized, a technical term coined for this production process, the required high temperatures destroy all of the live enzymes, beneficial bacteria, and even some of the vitamins and minerals. What is left is a product that has been associated with arthritis, digestive dysfunctions and cancer. In its raw and most natural form, however, milk comes from cows fed on grass, yielding a product higher in essential fatty acids than milk coming from dairy cows fed grain-dominated diets. Raw milk is full of beneficial vitamins and minerals and contains bacteria that help keep your digestive system healthy. Additionally, consumed in its raw form, the live enzymes in the milk—namely lactase— actually assist with the digestive process. This is why many people who think they are lactose-intolerant can consume raw milk with no ill effects. The milk has enzymes inside of it that help digest itself, creating less of a burden on your gut.

On the other hand, some foods are less healthy when overcooked. For example, meat that has been prepared with a crispy blackened layer contains high amounts of carcinogenic substances known as heterocyclic amines, or HCAs. While your body has the ability to handle these substances in small amounts, it's best to eat good quality meat cooked rare or medium rare and on a lower heat to preserve the enzymes and nutrients within it. It's also important to choose non-processed meats that don't have preservatives and additives in them that may increase shelf life but have been shown to be detrimental to your health. Just like any other food group, the less processing that goes into the food, the healthier it will be when you consume it.

The main consideration in both rare (or raw) meat and dairy is to choose the best quality product from the safest sources. For these two food groups, that means choosing organic meat and milk products from trusted sources—preferably local—from animals that were humanely treated. The importance of this consumer decision stretches far beyond personal health (see *Truly Sustainable Living*). It's not just meat though; the same is true for every food group. Quality matters.

Still other foods have benefits from being consumed raw or cooked, so eat both. Vegetables fall into this category. Eating fresh, organic vegetables will increase the vitamins and micronutrients in your diet, adding vital phytonutrients, antioxidants and vitamins that promote health and fight disease. But this doesn't mean that eating only raw vegetables is the answer. Cooking vegetables can also provide advantages. Many vegetables' vitamins and minerals are embedded in cellulose, a complex mass of fiber that is difficult to digest. In some cases, many of the nutrients in raw vegetables are not absorbed at all when consumed. Steaming or blanching the veggies will break these fibers down and make it easier on your digestive system.

If food is not digested properly, the macronutrients, vitamins and minerals will not be absorbed properly either. Digestion and absorption must happen in order for your body to take full advantage of any food, and cooking helps. When we heat, soften and moisturize vegetables during the cooking process, we dramatically increase the potential digestibility and absorption of many beneficial and nutritious compounds. More importantly, cooking can destroy some of the harmful anti-nutrients that bind minerals in the gut and interfere with the utilization of nutrients. Destruction of these anti-nutrients increases absorption and nutritional benefits.

Finally, some foods require careful and timely preparation methods. For example, many grains only reach their full health potential when they sprout, which effectively minimizes the adverse qualities commonly associated with many grain grain-based products. Therefore, choose breads and grain products that have been made from sprouted grains. Similarly, many legumes need to be soaked—sometimes several times—in order to disable toxins so they can be safely consumed without creating digestive responses that may be funny, but irritate the gut and cause inflammation. Fermented foods are yet another type of food which falls into this category. These digestion-improving foods have been through a process of lacto-fermentation, which is a process that preserves the food and creates beneficial enzymes, B-vitamins, Omega-3 fatty acids, and various strains of probiotics. That is why fermented foods like sauerkraut and kombucha have become recent health crazes.

The point, yet again, is that diversity matters. Some foods should be eaten raw, some should be cooked, and some should be soaked, sprouted, or fermented before consumption. These are not the only consumption options available to you, though. These are only a few that are important as you begin our journey of healthy eating.

When you ask *'How was it prepared?'* you get the conclusion of your food story. Each question—*What is it? Where did it come from? How was it prepared?*—creates a deeper storyline full of details you probably never thought you could get from a piece of food. More importantly, you learned something you can take with you as you can continue to make guided and informed decisions about your food and health. It gets easier and quicker each time you practice, so use these three questions until identifying real food becomes intuitive and instinctive.

Just... Eat... Real... Food.

This concept is so important that it requires revisiting. Real food—whole, unprocessed, unrefined, natural, organic—is superior to its counterpart. The reasons for this, while well documented and steeped in common sense, are still largely unknown. We still don't know everything there is to know in the real food world. The more we learn and deeper we go, the more questions we find. But what we do know is that if the health benefits of food only came down to the nutrients that were in it, ingesting extracts, fortifications and nutritional supplements would be just as good for you, if not better, than consuming the whole food from which they were derived. But this is not the case. Over and over again, studies show that the bioavailability of nutrient extracts does not match up to their whole food equivalents.[56] Broccoli extract is simply not as usable to the body as broccoli in its vegetable form.[57] The intrinsic qualities of food—the complexities we don't yet fully understand—make nature's originals far better than any extract or substitute that can be replicated in a lab.

There are many other confirmed reasons to choose whole food:

- Real food has more essential vitamins and minerals than processed food. Nutrient density makes the food healthier for the body.
- Real food is typically high in fiber and water than its processed counterparts, which means you will eat less and feel more satiated from the meal.[58]
- Real food is free of the chemicals and additives that make you feel like you need to eat more to satisfy your hunger. That hunger is not a real physiological need. It is simply a trick the additives in your food are playing on you. Once digested, the body metabolizes real food more efficiently and effectively, making it the superior choice for weight loss and management.[59]
- Real food is the best diet for your health because your body evolved to eat real food.[60] It's what your body needs to thrive.
- But the most important reason to eat real food is that it simply tastes better. Way better.

When you eat a diverse range of whole foods, variables like cholesterol, sodium, and sugar become largely redundant since whole food just doesn't contain unhealthy amounts of these substances. This diverse diet of whole real foods is also the formula for disease prevention, so you can scratch that off your list of things to worry about as well. This is why health food advocates proclaim that true healthcare reform starts in the kitchen.

Once you've made the switch to real food, track how many times you get sick in a year. Chances are you won't need to visit a doctor as much, thanks to your new and improved immune system.[32] In the end, eating real food means stressing less and focusing on the things that really matter. In the case of healthy eating, that's simply identifying real food.

The process of healthy living starts with a questioning and curious mind willing to ignore things at their face value and dig deeper for the real story. You are becoming a food detective, and with your health on the line, it will be time well spent.

Healthy Habits: Real Food

Food serves many purposes. Obviously it tastes good and makes you happy, but it also provides the raw goodness you need to rebuild your constantly changing physiology, deliver essential nutrients required for normal bodily chemical reactions, and make available the energy you need to function every single day of your life. No single food provides every single thing you need though. That's why you need a diverse range of foods from a variety of food groups prepared in different ways.

But there's a second part to this equation that we've ignored until now: biochemical individuality. It might be odd to think that so far we've paid no attention to specific food recommendations in a chapter that's all about food, but the truth is that we're all different, even when it comes to nutrition. For example, depending on a single gene, coffee can either prevent or promote heart disease.[61] Even a person's risk for disease resulting from insufficient or excessive amounts of salt consumption often depends on biochemical individuality. One person's food can be another person's poison, and it depends largely on the physiological factors that make us unique, namely genetics. Just as we all have different anatomical and physiological variations, we also have different responses to food and therefore unique nutritional requirements for optimal body function. These nutritional demands depend on our personal lifestyle choices and goals, such as our frequency and intensity of exercise, and desire to gain or lose weight.

Based on all of that, the only person who can decide if a certain food is healthy or not is … you. Ignore the marketing and hype. Listen to your body. What is it telling you? There's an innate and profound wisdom in the body that people do not listen to anymore—or simply can't hear any more. They seek answers from external sources instead of establishing the connection with their own body. The body doesn't lie. With practice and a little effort, you will become your own nutritional guru. The process starts when you begin implementing healthy habits that reconnect you with the entire food experience. The healthy eating habits provided below serve to empower you and your dietary practices.

1. Kitchen Makeover

Before you can effectively embark on a total health makeover, your kitchen needs one too. If you want a healthy lifestyle, and especially a healthy diet, surround yourself with healthy choices. Keeping ice cream, potato chips and chocolate bars in the refrigerator is a surefire way to sabotage your progress. And let's face it, if there are snacks in the house, they're going to get eaten. It's only a matter of time.

Start off by throwing away any food from your pantry and refrigerator that's unhealthy. If you know it's not real food, toss it. If you have to sit and think about whether a certain food item qualifies as real food, it doesn't. Toss it. It's not that you'll never eat these foods again, it's just that you need to get them out of your house to help prevent emotional eating binges. When you're at home, healthy choices need to be convenient and unhealthy choices inconvenient. If you find yourself craving unhealthy foods, you will have to go out of your way and buy them. This small hurdle could be the difference between making a healthy or an unhealthy food choice.

Open your pantry. Take out all the bad stuff. Toss it. Open your fridge. Repeat the same steps. You're welcome.

2. Keep a Food Journal

The truth is that most people think they already eat pretty well. They'll tell you all about the healthy choices they make on a daily basis, but studies show that people don't accurately measure their food intakes.[62] The problem is people 'forget' the bad nutritional choices they make or simply choose to ignore them. Why would anyone make themselves look bad in a conversation about eating habits? They wouldn't. They forget they ate that chocolate bar when they were bored. They ignore the sugar-filled latte from the coffee shop they had as a mid-morning snack. *They don't count, right?*

Here's where food journaling can help: becoming aware of food choices, tracking feedback and responses from certain foods, and planning meals. Self-monitoring food choices, logging those choices, and planning meals with a food journal provides a strategy that's proven to be beneficial for weight management and getting healthier.[63]

Food Choice Awareness

Most people just don't think about what they put in their mouths. The best way to become more conscious of everything you put into your body is to write it all down and track it. When you start journaling what you eat, you'll think twice about that candy bar if you know it will forever be inked into your journal. Becoming aware of your food choices is the first step to healthy eating. It's the starting point of reconnecting with your body.

Physiological Feedback

Your food journal is also a tool that will help you tap into your own responses and reactions to food and keep track of the diversity of your diet. Only by bringing awareness to your food choices and documenting them will you be able to find the best food formula for your unique body. *What do I eat or drink that makes me feel best before workouts? After workouts? What do I eat to make sure I sleep well at night? At what time? Have I had enough fruits and vegetables today? Why am I always hungry at 3pm?* All of these questions can be answered by documenting your food choices, trial-and-error experimenting and researching the issue for yourself.

Meal Planning

Give yourself a real head-start on your healthier life by planning your meals in advance. Why? So you don't have to stress out about what you're going to eat next; your healthy options are already planned out for you. Time meals effectively, cater for functional meals like pre- or post-exercise nutrition, and schedule dietary diversity into your meals.

Let's face it. Your default meal-on-the-run is probably something that's convenient and fast, possibly takeout or fast food. But if you don't have to waste time or energy deciding what to eat because you've already planned ahead, all you have to do is follow the directions you've created for yourself.

Planning your meals also means planning your grocery shopping in advance. Make your shopping trips more efficient and cheaper by listing all the meals you're going to cook at home for the week then creating an ingredients list. You'll also waste less food in the process. See? It's quick, easy and efficient.

3. Conscious Consumption

One of the conveniences of our modern world is that food is readily available at a moment's notice. But this convenience has spiraled out of control thanks to the worst concept to ever hit mainstream American culture: the all-you-can-eat buffet. There's absolutely no need to exploit this convenience and stuff yourself every time you sit down to eat. Overeating can be stressful to your digestive system and adversely impact your health. Just like you need a holiday every now and again, your digestive system sometimes needs a break, too.

Bring consciousness back to an unconscious act. At midday, instead of wolfing down your lunch and thinking about those 14 unread emails blinking at you from your inbox or that afternoon meeting you really don't want to go to, bring your focus back to the food you're putting in your mouth. Mentally stepping away from everything else and really paying attention to your food can help you satisfy your hunger without overeating. Try these tools to reconnect with your body and make eating a mindful—rather than mindless—activity:

- Hara Hachi Bu, an ancient Confucian philosophy, teaches people to eat until they are 80% satisfied. Reconnect with your body and consciously stop eating when you feel 80% full.

- Take two big diaphragmatic breaths between bites. These big breathes give you an opportunity to assess satiety. They also help to relax your body by activating your parasympathetic nervous system, thus aiding the digestive process.
- Chew each bite of food at least 20 times before swallowing. Thorough mastication allows a greater surface area of your food to be covered with saliva, which allows digestive enzymes to start the demanding task of breaking down foods into absorbable forms. Munching more will lower the stress applied to your stomach, allow more nutrients from your meal to be absorbed, and provide your digestive system with a little more time to send satiety hormones to the brain to tell it when you're full.

With each of these practices, you're intently listening to your body and slowing down when you eat. Pick the approach that best fits your personality, then stick to it. Ultimately, the goal is to prevent overeating while providing your body with the fuel it needs to function. Hunger is not a state of mind that should be feared; constant satiety should. Ironically, hunger has been shown to improve productivity and sharpen cognitive function;[64] and research has shown that brief periods of fasting can significantly strength immune function and rejuvenate the body.[65] By eating less, you'll live longer,[66,67] but that doesn't imply starvation.[68] It simply means eating healthy food, mindfully. The more tuned into your body you are, the more sustainable your healthy eating habits will be.

4. Eat Real Food

Armed with the three questions for identifying real food—*What is it? Where did it come from? How was it prepared?*—eat a diet focused predominantly on whole, and natural food. To help you further with mealtime selections, here are some helpful guidelines.

Eat Vegetables at Every Meal

The healthiest foods that will have the greatest and most immediate impact on your health and wellbeing are vegetables. Eat them at every meal. Pick different ones and explore as many options as you can. The more diverse your selection, the better.

Eat Protein at Every Meal

One of the recent nutritional myths sweeping across the country is that eating too much protein can harm your health by putting excessive strain on the kidneys and damaging your bones. Both of these notions have been proven to be false.[69,70,71] Most alarming is that people hear this kind of sensationalist media and stop eating protein altogether. This could be a huge mistake if you're trying to get healthy.

While you might associate protein with muscle-building activities—of course, it does work that way—you can also use proteins to help manage your blood sugar levels. Protein is known to be useful to your body by making it easier to keep your blood sugar levels in check. Much of this benefit comes from the development of amino acids to help you control how your body handles sugar. Amino acids are essential for promoting muscle growth, which in return makes you stronger and more likely to live a healthy life without all those sugar cravings.[72]

Protein improves your metabolism, curbs hunger, reduces your risk of diabetes,[73] and provides the raw materials you need for organ support and lean muscle maintenance.[74] In fact, protein is a component of every cell in your body.

Dietary protein comes from a variety of sources, including

meat, fish, eggs, dairy or legumes. Include one of these protein sources with every meal.

Don't Be Scared of Healthy Fat

Despite popular opinion, eating fat will not make you fat. In fact, the opposite has been shown to be true.[75,76] This doesn't mean you should only eat fat, but it does mean that fat has a very important place in a healthy diet and shouldn't be demonized, particularly saturated fat and its relationship with the heart. We've all heard the claims that saturated fat consumption directly increases heart disease however these claims have been refuted.[77,78] A meta-analysis of 347,747 subjects showed no significant evidence that dietary saturated fat is directly associated with an increased risk of heart disease.[79]

Simply put, dietary fat is essential for the human body to function. It provides energy for human functions, is required for healthy hormone production, necessary for vitamin absorption, and critical for hair and skin health. Healthy, unprocessed, and natural fats like **coconut oil, avocado, fish, butter, nuts, seeds and animal products** are all useful for your body's needs.

Smart Carbs

Excessive consumption of processed sugar can have severe adverse health implications, including rapid weight gain,[80] metabolic disease,[81] and a host of chronic diseases like obesity,[82] heart disease[83] and type 2 diabetes.[84,85] Furthermore, sugar does not create satiety; in fact it often creates the desire to eat more.[86] This applies to fructose from added sugars, not the natural sugars found in foods like fruit, which are a healthy part of a diverse diet.

People eat too many carbohydrates, especially in the form of refined and processed sugars. White bread, pasta, sugary snacks, candy, soft drinks, fruit juice, soda, breakfast cereals, salad dressings, sweet condiments, sauces and alcohol are all common sources of unnecessary sugars that have little to no nutritional value. These foods simply do not provide the micronutrients, vitamins, and minerals the body needs to thrive.

Don't eliminate all carbohydrates from your diet, though. Carbs are an extremely important part of a healthy diet and—when consumed and timed for a specific functional need—they can be highly advantageous. For example, eating carbohydrates after intense exercise assists your body with the recovery process. Lots of variables determine the amount of carbs an individual should be eating, but the main ones to consider are daily movement level and fitness and weight loss goals. The more you move, the more carbohydrates you need.

When it comes to carbs, however, it's important to consume 'smart carbs'. Carbohydrates from **fruits, vegetables, whole grains and legumes** are superior to processed and manufactured alternatives.

Real Food Cheat Sheet

Food Group	Best Choice	Worst Choice
Vegetables	Fermented, Non-GMO, Organic, Local	Canned
Meat & Fish	Organic, Local, Grass-fed, Wild-caught	Processed, Cured, Overcooked
Fruit	Fresh, Frozen, Organic, Local	Canned, Dried, Juice, Jellies, Jams, Candied
Legumes	Organic, Soaked	Canned, Processed, Soy
Nuts	Sprouted, Raw, Roasted	Salted
Dairy	Raw	Pasteurized
Grain	Sprouted, Whole	White

To make the process easier to digest and to provide a useful resource to quickly reference in times of confusion, provided on the previous page is a Real Food reference chart that shows the best and worst sources and preparation methods for the various food groups. Use it as necessary.

5. Ditch the Liquid Calories

The only liquid your body needs is the most important micronutrient for life: water. There are certainly health benefits associated with varieties of herbal teas and quality coffee, but in terms of necessity, it's water that your body craves and requires for optimal function.

Ditch the sugary beverages that provide no nutritional value and make you unhealthy like soda, fruit juice and energy drinks. [87,88,89] You can put alcohol on this list as well, depending on how serious you are about your health goals. If we're being honest though, the more you drink, the harder it will be to meet your health goals.

But liquid calories aren't just limited to your favorite cheat drink; they also include dressings, sauces, and condiments that can turn regular meals into junk food. You can actually can make healthy dressings and sauces with a few simple and healthy ingredients that will taste better and be far healthier than the ones you currently use.

6. Reconnect with the Food Experience

People have lost connection with their food, where it comes from, and the amount of knowledge involved in growing healthy food. This isn't surprising considering that the only connection an individual may have with the food production system is the end result: seeing aisles of neatly packaged food products inside a grocery store. We typically don't see what's going on in the kitchen, much less what happened in a farmer's field or in on an assembly line, so we passively accept what is put on our plates.

The obvious way to reconnect with the food experience is to meet your food producers and farmers in order to establish a relationship and gain an understanding of what is involved in the production of healthy food. Growing your own food is another option. Nutritional knowledge, attitudes about healthy eating and environmental responsibility, and eating behaviors all improve when an individual is involved and invested in the educational process of growing food.[90]

For many, however, growing their own food is simply not possible. The lifestyle demands and environmental considerations of modern day people living in urban areas make it difficult to find the time and space for garden upkeep. Luckily, food production is only one of the ways of reconnecting with the food experience.

Cultivate Culinary Creativity

The three questions for identifying real food and reconnecting with the entire food experience are *what is it, where did it come from, and how was it prepared.* The only way to have full control over all three variables is to take the spatula into your own hands and prepare the food yourself. When you cook, you get to choose the ingredients and the cooking methods yourself. You get a firsthand experience with the story of each food you select and the ability to create a narrative pleasing to the palate. It's time to get in touch with your inner chef.

You don't have to go to an expensive cooking school to learn how to cook in a healthy and delicious way. These days it's easier than ever to become a top-notch cook. Take classes at a local school. Get alongside a friend who has a knack in the kitchen.

Watch different television programs dedicated to teaching you how to cook. And of course, traditional cookbooks always help. You might be amazed at what you can do in the kitchen. Experiment with a wide range of natural herbs and spices to add as much healthiness to your dishes as flavor.

Just remember it takes time to refine your cooking skills, so if your broccoli turns into little chunks of charcoal, don't get discouraged. Try again. Every time you try a new dish, you get to play a little bit more creatively and learn as you fashion your culinary creation. The good news is that your friends will have no problem being taste-testers for your dishes. I haven't met anyone yet who would turn down a healthy home-cooked meal!

Make Eating a Social Experience
What's the point of cooking if you're not enjoying it with others? There is no greater pleasure than satisfying the taste buds and appetites of your friends and loved ones. Make it a habit to cook for someone at least once a week. Host potlucks and bring groups together to enjoy food the way it was meant to be enjoyed. Food is an experience that's better shared in the company of others. It's slow rather than fast, social rather than solitary, and fun rather than monotonous. You'll learn new things, foster and grow relationships, and enjoy one of the neglected simple pleasures of life—just hanging out with people.

When you make eating a social activity, remember something very important. Your friends have a greater impact on your health than you think. You've probably heard the adage before that you are the five people you spend the most time with you. That is especially true for your health. If you have obese and unhealthy friends, you are more likely to be obese or unhealthy yourself.[91,92] If your friends are unhealthy, it may be time to find new ones.

Eat with Gratitude

The longer you maintain healthy eating habits, the more you realize healthy eating is more about *how* you eat, not *what* you eat. Your emotional state of being significantly influences what you choose to eat[93] and how that food is digested. Be calm, peaceful and eat in a state of gratitude, and your wellbeing will improve across several different aspects of your life.[94] Your mindset before, during and after eating will impact your digestive, biochemical and hormonal systems, so make sure you remain thankful for the meal in front of you.[95] A peaceful and calm attitude of gratitude will ensure proper digestive function.[96]

...

What happens when you're not at home being the king of your own consumption? Well, the truth is you won't always be surrounded by the healthiest food options. The object of the game is not to be perfect, but rather to do the best you can with what you've got. If you're traveling, eating out with friends or at a work function, simply weigh up the options in front of you and work with them rather than stressing about perfection. Your routine will be ready for you the next day, and it's better to enjoy the present moment than stress and complain about it. Accept the situation for what it is and just have fun.

Above all else, remember that you're not perfect. Neither is your diet. Don't judge others for their dietary choices if they don't think the same way as you. If someone asks about yours or you ask about theirs, start with the points you both agree on then move on from there. Keep it friendly. Arguing and passionately defending your food choices gets you nowhere fast. But if you politely chat and agree to disagree, you may come away with a bit of information or perspective you didn't have before and be smarter for it. There is no one right way to live. There never has been, and there never will be. There are a million ways to live.

Movement

"Worms will not eat living wood where the vital sap is flowing; rust will not hinder the opening of a gate when the hinges are used each day. Movement gives health and life. Stagnation brings disease and death."
– Ancient Chinese Proverb

"Yes, exercise is the catalyst. That's what makes everything happen: your digestion, your elimination, your sex life, your skin, hair, everything about you depends on circulation. And how do you increase circulation?" – Jack LaLanne

Next up on the Lifestyle Transformation checklist is movement and exercise. To be perfectly honest, exercise hasn't been very high on David's priority list for quite some time now. He gets winded just walking from his car to the office——and he parks in the same building. Given his lack of experience on the fitness front, David knows he could do with all the help he can get. He books a session with a personal trainer where he confides his greatest fear and why he's looking for a nudge in the right direction:

My grandfather was in a wheelchair for the last years of his life. I saw how difficult it was for him, how it trapped him, how he was forced to give up his independence. He used to be very active when he was younger. He loved running. He just loved doing stuff. To see how his energy, demeanor and personality deteriorated almost immediately is something I'll never forget. The only advice he gave me was to never take my ability to move for granted. Always keep moving. That's what he really wanted me to understand——I guess so I didn't end up like him. So that's why I'm here. I want to keep moving for the rest of my life. I don't want to end up in a wheelchair like my grandfather.

The fitness trainer nods empathetically all the while taking notes. He understands David's fears, but he needs to go deeper, to find out more about how he lives day to day. He asks for a 'Day in the Life of David' in order to understand how much movement he currently gets. David describes his typical day:

I wake up at 7am, and usually spend 15 minutes in bed before finally getting up to get dressed. I sit down to eat breakfast for 15 minutes, rush out the door and spend 60 minutes in traffic commuting to work. I have a computer job, so I spend roughly nine hours in my cubicle at my desk. I only get up briefly to go to the bathroom, grab a quick meal (which I eat at my desk), or brew a cup of coffee. I spend another 60 minutes in traffic on the way home. My evening usually consists of three hours watching TV on the couch and another hour on my laptop browsing the internet for articles, videos or checking email. I squeeze my dinner into that time since I eat while watching my favorite shows. Finally, I sleep for eight hours ... then do it all again the following day.

David's trainer slowly looks up from his notes with a grim look on his face. He pauses before speaking. *David, do you realize that you're already living in a wheelchair, just like your grandfather?* David is confused. *What do you mean?* David's trainer calmly states that he spends 23 ½ hours of the day either sitting or lying down—that's just 30 minutes where he gets up and moves around. David wants to avoid the confined and dependent life his grandfather was forced to endure yet he's already unknowingly living it. He's robbing himself of the ability to move around freely and independently the older he gets by living the kind of sedentary lifestyle that's more common today than it's ever been at any other point in human history.

Sitting Kills. Movement Heals.

Sometimes we don't realize just how amazing the human body really is. It withstands all of the forces, demands and stresses placed on it then does something truly incredible: it adapts to them. When you gaze at Cirque de Soleil contortionists bend and twist beyond belief, behold superhuman feats of strength, or sit in awe as professional athletes practically defy the laws of physics right before your eyes, you are witnessing the combined force of countless tiny adaptations of your body that eventually led to that single incredible moment.

But feats of this caliber do not happen accidentally. What we often forget is the ongoing training, the trial and error, the discipline and practice, right down to the tiny innate steps the body takes every single day that lead to these kinds of memorable and awe-inspiring moments. They're the result of a mindful and intentional process—a process that's happening to all of us every waking moment whether you are aware of it or not. Your body constantly adapts to the way you live your life. And that's a major problem if you live a predominantly sedentary lifestyle.

It doesn't take a rocket scientist to figure out that if you lift enough weight, you'll probably build muscle. The reverse is also very true. If you remove movement and exercise from your life, your body will adapt to that, too. Did you know that astronauts returning home from the final frontier have to be taken off the shuttle in wheelchairs? While they're outside Earth's stratosphere, their bodies adapt to the lack of gravitational forces with weaker and more brittle bones.[1] If they attempt to walk out on their own when they return to Earth, they could actually fracture or break their own bones. This adaptation is not a sign of weakness; in fact, it's quite the opposite. It actually illustrates the body's capability to adapt to the most extreme of environments. You don't need bone density in space because gravity doesn't smash down on you 24 hours a day when you're on a space station. As a result, your body adapts to zero gravity by reallocating those precious biological resources normally needed for bone density maintenance to other functions that are far more useful in outer space.

Similarly, the innate ability to adapt to external force and pressure also explains why sitting for long periods of time can be very harmful to our bodies. When our bodies adapt to an inactive sedentary lifestyle, they do so in many ways. Structurally speaking, the first adaptation of a sedentary lifestyle is muscular atrophy. As the old adage goes, use it or lose it. Muscles become weaker since the body assumes they're just not needed—just like an astronaut doesn't need strong bones in space. Biological resources normally used in muscle development and maintenance are used elsewhere in the body, resulting in weaker, smaller and flabbier muscles. In turn, this creates joint instability, an increased likelihood of injury, and decreased circulation of vital oxygen and nutrients.[2] Take a look at your glutes. The longer you sit, the flatter and weaker your glutes will get. You can literally deflate your derrière if your lifestyle is dominated by sitting. While this may seem like a strictly aesthetic problem, atrophied and dysfunctional hips can be major contributors to hip and lower back problems.

Sitting also causes some muscles and connective tissue to shorten, because muscles can't express their full range of motion during normal everyday activity. This is why many people often complain of feeling 'tight' after sitting too long. Shortened muscles influence joint angles, which in turn impact posture and alignment. Specifically, sitting shortens and tightens hip flexor muscles, which can create strain on the lower back. Over time, this adaptation can cause long-term changes to the alignment of your pelvis, including a forward tilt that makes you look like you're sticking your butt out like Jennifer Lopez. While this might be appropriate in the Las Vegas club scene, this structural deviation adversely impacts your bodily function. Not only will standing upright become more energetically taxing on the body, but the forces generated by walking and running will force joints, tendons, and ligaments to move in nonfunctional ways, often resulting in chronic aches and pains. The altered position of the pelvis means the body simply doesn't absorb gravitational forces the way it was designed to.

Lastly, sitting impacts the connective tissue and collagen fibers that run throughout the body, commonly referred to as fascia. When we hold our bodies in any position, the body adapts by making that area tight so muscles are not overworked in the process. It's a brilliant way to conserve precious energy. When we sit, the muscles and fascia of the lower back adapt by stiffening, thus making the lower back immobile and inflexible. While this conserves energy and protects the muscles of the lower back from being overworked, it reduces your range of motion, creates stiffness and increases the likelihood of injury.[3] The longer you sit and the longer your lifestyle remains sedentary, the more 'glued' together these areas become. Your fascia simply responds to the adaptations—or lack thereof—placed on it. In turn, the longer your body is stuck, the more difficult it becomes to undo this process. No longer being able to bend over and touch your toes doesn't just come down to inflexibility; in truth a series of small adaptations over a long period of time led to this state of inflexibility. Your body adapted to sitting—and that's definitely not good for your health.

Next time you watch toddlers move around, appreciate their wonderful displays of flexibility, mobility and range of motion with every movement, especially squatting down. If you don't have children, watch cats and dogs stretch when they wake up from sleep. They move around and express their mobility regularly so they don't lose it. Even though this is an instinctive behavior, it should still illustrate the point. You once had these movement abilities, too. They were not lost overnight. It took years of small adaptations as your body simply adjusted to the movement requirements—or lack thereof—placed on it. If nothing in your lifestyle demands the ability to squat, then that ability will be lost.

The more you sit, the better your body becomes at sitting. That might be fine for a typical day of waking up, going to work and coming home, only to repeat it all again the next day, but what happens when life throws you a curveball? What happens when you slip, trip or fall? If your body has totally adapted to sitting, it won't be prepared to contort, reach, stretch and brace itself as it attempts to deal with unexpected physical requirements. You might break a bone, sprain a joint, tear a muscle or put your back out because your body isn't prepared for the unexpected situations life throws at you. If you've ever been injured you'll understand the torture of not being able to move pain-free. It can sometimes lead to depression, but it's also a surefire way to learn never to take the independence movement gives you for granted. Unfortunately, an injury is often the wake-up call that finally makes us realize that we've taken our movement for granted.

It's not just our muscles that atrophy from the lack of movement; the consequences of a sedentary lifestyle also impact us on a biological level. An inactive lifestyle can cause metabolic changes that adversely affect triglycerides, cholesterol, blood sugar and blood pressure. In other words, your entire body begins to atrophy from the inside out, increasing your chances of chronic conditions like obesity, metabolic syndrome, type 2 diabetes and cardiovascular disease.[4,5,6]

Humans were not designed for a sedentary lifestyle. While we're getting better at the task by adapting our structure to make sitting easier, our inactivity contributes to chronic health conditions that severely limit the quality of our daily lives. But remember that the body is an incredible—and fast—adapter to the demands we place on it. So if a sedentary lifestyle was the way that we got into the problem, the way out is self-explanatory: movement. If sitting kills, then movement heals.

The best way to prevent the ill effects of a sedentary lifestyle is to fight fire with fire. You have to get up and move. When you start moving and doing exercise on a regular basis, you immediately set in motion the biological and metabolic processes the body needs for healing. Movement and exercise strengthen and improve the immune system which makes the body better equipped to stave off disease.[7] Exercise also improves the immune system by boosting white blood cell performance and detoxifying through sweat. Every time you choose to move, you are effectively building up a defense against future illness and disease. This also helps explain why people who regularly exercise get sick less often and, when they do fall sick, for a shorter period of time.

Exercise also improves cognitive function. It enhances memory, improves learning capabilities, boosts attention span, and even improves decision-making because of its impact on important brain neurotransmitters like dopamine, serotonin, and norepinephrine. Exercise makes the brain more adaptive and assists in reorganizing neural pathways based on new experiences. This is why the most creative souls throughout time made it a point to move. It was in these moments of movement that their greatest creations came to fruition.

Regular exercise also impacts the other kind of movement. Bowel movements become more regular thanks to increased blood flow throughout your digestive system, as well as the natural pressure your internal organs receive when your movements create contractions around the intestines. Exercise is also one of the best ways to manage stress, providing a healthy outlet for stressful situations, all the while lowering every cardiometabolic risk factor across the board.[8] Exercise is your fountain of youth and the most potent anti-aging therapy available.[9,10] The secret to life is simple. Just keep moving.

Movement heals. It's a saying most people have heard but few fundamentally understand, but it has everything to do with circulation. When you get enough movement during the day, your muscles act as biological pumps that help your heart propel water, oxygen and nutrients around your body, creating all of the health benefits discussed previously and more. You will simply feel great every time you move.

Humans evolved to move. Emotionally, movement reduces levels of anxiety and depression.[11,12] Mentally, it instantly improves cognitive function and learning capabilities.[13] Psychologically, it provides an efficient and effective way of managing stress.[14] These benefits hold true even if you are forced to exercise against your will.[15] Structurally, it maintains or improves bone density and lean muscle tissue.[16,17,18,19] Energetically, it clears blocked energy pathways and calms the mind. Digestively, it lowers the burden placed on your intestines by helping to keep bowel movements regular.[20] And in terms of circulation, it assists the heart in pumping oxygen and nutrients throughout your body while simultaneously detoxing your body by removing waste through the lymphatic system.[21] We need movement. Everyday. And often.

Strength + Flexibility = Power = Longevity

For some people, the term 'exercise' provokes feelings of excitement, adrenalin and anticipation. For others, the word brings with it intimidation, apprehension and fear. The beauty of exercise, though, is that no single form of exercise works for everyone and there's no one right way of doing it. On one hand, that can be daunting; where do you even start? On the other hand, it's incredibly liberating. Nike was onto something when they exclaimed 'Just do it!' Just have a go at something—anything. Experiment with a range of different activities and forms of exercise. Don't worry if you decide cycling isn't really for you after all; just try something else. However, if you're looking for longevity it's important to create a balanced movement and exercise strategy in order to get the most out of it and keep your body safe while doing it. To understand these exercise objectives, understand this analogy of the slingshot first.

As a child, you would load a slingshot with something small like a stone, pull the rubber band back as far as it would go, close your eyes, grit your teeth, let it go, and pray your stone made it further than the other kids'. For your stone to reach its maximum distance and force potential, though, a number of elements had to work in sync. There's the frame, the foundation of the slingshot. If it's weak or worn, pulling back on the band could break the frame off at its base. Then there's the band itself. Firstly it needs maximum stretch. The farther the band can stretch, the more power and distance will be behind the shot. If you can only pull the band back a little bit, it doesn't matter how strong you or the frame are or how new the rubber is, the stone will not travel far or powerfully. Secondly, the band needs to be in good condition. If it's worn, cracked or dried out, the band could snap when it's stretched back or go limp because it lacks the elasticity to snap back to its original shape. The more the frame and band are cared for, the longer the slingshot will be able to powerfully fire stones through the air. This is like the delicate balance of your body's strength and flexibility.

Strength

Just like the slingshot, a strong underlying framework gives your body the stability it needs to move through its full range of motion successfully and safely. To create a strong bodily framework, regular movement and exercise is essential to trigger your body's growth and repair response that builds muscle, increases metabolism and makes you stronger. In turn, these physiological adaptations give you independence. You can pick up your children. You can carry your own groceries in from the car. You can walk up stairs and hike up mountains. Strength lets you do what you want when you want, without limitation. Strength is freedom.

As we discovered earlier, sedentary lifestyles can result in harmful effects on hip function, so it's important to pay special attention to strengthening and developing the glutes. It might sound weird, but nothing is more functional than regularly training your butt. Your glutes are (supposed to be) the strongest muscles in your body. Their anatomical position and size have evolved over time to allow the human body to lift its forelimbs off the ground.[22] When we ask the much smaller and inefficient muscles of the lower back to do work designed for the glutes, like lifting heavy objects off the ground, they are placed in a vulnerable position which increases the chance of lower back injury. This is why people with lumbar problems often have stronger lower backs than those with healthy backs. The tiny weaker muscles of the lower back are worked more intensely while the stronger and all-important glutes are largely ignored. Strengthening these tiny muscles can only do so much since they are so small to begin with. Their potential for strength development is limited.

The glutes, on the other hand, are big muscles with big strength potential. They're the largest muscles in your body and are designed—based on both physiological position and orientation—to do all that heavy lifting the lower back just shouldn't be asked to do. Developing glute strength and functionality may be the most proactive step you can take to protecting your lower back. Don't be scared of exercises like squats, deadlifts or lunges; your glutes are very capable muscles and need to be pushed beyond their capacity in order to develop and adapt. Look at your glutes as your supporting cast that will strengthen and complement all of the movement and exercise activities you choose to do. Without strong glutes, you put unnecessary and excessive pressure on the rest of your body.

From yoga practice and improving running form and endurance, to walking up stairs or simply playing with your kids, strength training will make your life easier and help you feel more capable. As you age, a strong and capable body will keep you vibrant and vital, and help you maintain your freedom for longer.

Flexibility

Flexibility is not about doing the splits; it's actually about moving the various joints of your body through their optimal range of motion freely and painlessly. Optimum flexibility helps prevent aches, pains and injuries, and lets you feel free, open and confident from the inside out. It enables you to perform everyday activities like getting out of bed, reaching for objects, or sweeping the floor with ease. Flexibility is your body's ability to creatively express itself. Never lose that ability to move freely.

Many people think that how far a muscle can be stretched is a reflection of flexibility. That is true, but it's only half of the equation. Flexibility is comprised of two variables: tissue extensibility and joint mobility. The amount of stretch a muscle can withstand is commonly called tissue extensibility. This has to do with how far your hamstring or chest muscles can be stretched, or how far the band on your slingshot can be pulled back. Tissue extensibility, is more than just an assessment of the muscle itself. While the muscle length is important, so too is the quality and health of the fascia, the connective tissue enveloping and surrounding the muscle. Not only does fascia adapt to physical demands like sitting they're also influenced by other factors that many of us don't realize. Dehydration, inflammation caused by poor food choices like excessive sugar consumption, and even mental or emotional factors can play a significant role in poor fascial health. For example, if you create inflammation with an unhealthy diet, your flexibility will be impaired as well. If you feel depressed, your posture will slump. Improving and maintaining tissue extensibility is an integrative process that's more than just stretching regularly. It requires a holistic and comprehensive approach to your health and wellbeing.

The second aspect of flexibility focuses on where the muscles originate from: the joints. It doesn't matter how stretchy your muscles might naturally be if your joints have become 'stuck' or adapted to an immobile environment like sitting. If your joint mobility is limited, your muscles can't stretch as far as they'd normally be able to. **Our ankles, hips and thoracic spine are the primary areas affected by modern sedentary lifestyles, yet healthy ankles, hips and backs are essential for a lifetime of free and easy movement.**

Without exception, every movement and exercise strategy should address these major joints because deficiencies in any one of them can lead to detrimental side effects. Ankle mobility issues can cause chronic knee and hip pain. Hip immobility can lead to knee pain or lower back pain. Thoracic spine immobility can lead to lower back pain, neck pain, or even shoulder injuries. Mobility is nobility. Optimal mobility at the major joints of the body—ankles, hips, and thoracic spine—creates the potential for lifelong healthy movement.

Power = Longevity

Just like a slingshot, optimal human function is determined by the ability to produce power. In the human body this is a unique display of strength through an optimal range of motion, done very quickly. If you want to increase your power, you need both strength and flexibility equally. Neither characteristic is more important than the other since they both need to work together to create the foundation for longevity. You need balance.

Let's look at the application of power and how it translates into longevity. Imagine tripping over a small object, jumping out of the way of an oncoming vehicle, or catching yourself with your arms to prevent a fall. While these situations don't happen every day, making sure your body is prepared for them is the difference between protecting and injuring yourself. In fact, falls like this are one of the leading causes of deaths in elderly populations. Do you know someone who was in perfectly fine health until an accident triggered a series of events that led them into serious illness? If the accident itself doesn't do it, the resulting lack of movement, independence and strength will restrict immune function and make the person more susceptible to illness. This is why power is important; you never know when you'll need it. Life always has unexpected twists and turns, and you need to be able to quickly mobilize and protect your body at a moment's notice. If your body is physically prepared to handle life's twists and turns, you will improve your likelihood of lifelong health and longevity.

Choosing where to start depends completely on the individual. If someone is very flexible and mobile but is inherently weak, then it's best to focus on developing strength through that range of motion. Otherwise, this would be equivalent to pulling the band of a slingshot back, letting go, and the slack band simply falling to the floor without any recoil. At the other end of the spectrum, if someone has all the strength in the world but limited mobility, it makes sense to focus on improving their range of motion to reduce the likelihood of injury should an accident require an increased range of motion or flexibility.

When you train specifically for power—that is, strength through an optimal range of motion as quickly as possible—you improve the sphere of potential motion within your body. Imagine you have an injured shoulder. Your sphere of potential motion is limited due to the pain you would experience in your shoulder should you attempt to lift or reach your arm out. The same is true if you have an extremely weak core. You can't reach as high or far because your core muscles can't support your bodyweight. Both strength and flexibility play important parts in your sphere of motion.

Movement is your gauge of health and your fountain of youth. If you started with little movement but find that your sphere of motion is growing, you're effectively reversing your age and getting younger. The greater your sphere of potential motion, the healthier you are.

Healthy Spine for a Healthy Life

Regardless of which type of exercise you choose to do, there are three fundamental qualities of movement that must be maintained in order to maintain maximum effectiveness and injury prevention: alignment, form and posture (AFP). (Since all three of these qualities must be considered with each and every movement, they will now be referred to as AFP.) AFP dictates which muscles fire and which joints are stressed, and plays an intricate part in injury prevention. According to scientific studies, wrong AFP is actually the top cause of injuries. To illustrate just how important AFP is to human function, let's examine the most basic of human functions: walking.

As we learnt earlier, human beings have evolved to move, not sit. Evolutionary adaptations have created structure and function that makes bipedal movement—walking and running—energy-efficient. It took millions of years for the human body to develop its upright standing posture, evolving biological mechanisms to battle the force of gravity. Today, human bodies actually utilize gravitational force for their benefit when they walk.

Confused? Imagine a spring resting on a table. You push down on the spring to 'load' it. When you let go, it releases all of its stored energy and pops up (be careful not to place your face too close to the spring though). Now let's apply this spring to everyday walking. Your body is the spring and gravity is the force pushing the spring down to load it. Every time you take a step, gravity pushes on you, in essence compressing you like a spring. Due to your various bone and joint alignments, muscle and tendon tensions, and directions of pull, this creates a 'loaded' spring effect that the body uses to propel you forward from step to step. Every time you step, gravity loads the spring once more and the release of energy creates forward momentum.

When you walk with correct AFP, these gravitational forces are absorbed and utilized by the body in a way that's not only safe but very energy efficient. Have you ever wondered why you can walk for several minutes—if not hours—at a time, yet only do 10 reps of moderately heavy biceps curls before your muscles give out? Human bipedal movement is the epitome of energy efficiency. Why fight the constant force of gravity when it can be used to help you move instead?

Walking is an energetically cheap task for the human body because you essentially use gravitational forces to load the springs of your body from step to step, and the release of energy is just your muscles being passively loaded by gravity. This efficiency is no accident. Evolution has provided the human body with the structure and underlying function it needs to get its hands on food without requiring too much energy. It's a high rate of return for a low investment and certainly one of the important reasons for our species' evolutionary success.

Now let's take a look at what the human body looks like when AFP is not appropriate. Imagine someone with a sedentary lifestyle. What does this person's posture look like? Rounded shoulders? Yes. Feet turned out? Most likely. Head slightly forward? Yup. With this misaligned frame, muscles are anatomically positioned to be inefficient, ligaments are strained, and decreased joint space prevents optimal range of motion from occurring at the shoulders and hips. Abnormal weight is gained around the abdomen and belly, and their glutes are flat, lazy and ineffective.

Now imagine this person walking. Take this misaligned frame

and allow it to absorb the constant forces of gravity hundreds—if not thousands—of times every day. Now imagine this frame running instead of walking, which creates vertical force that your body must absorb that is equal to as much as 2.5 times your body weight.[23]

This misaligned body can only withstand so many thousands of repetitions of walking and running before inflammation turns into pain which then can turn into a chronic injury. Any human body will break down under these conditions. Human bipedal movement was designed to absorb gravity in a specific way. The longer you deviate from this underlying function, the higher the likelihood of injury. How many runners do you know currently struggle with ankle, hip or knee pain? It's no secret that runners keep physical therapists in business.

If AFP matters with walking and running—the most basic of human movements—then it definitely applies to every other form of movement and exercise. When you exercise, AFP allows the right muscles to receive most of the forces. When you compensate and AFP deteriorates during exercise, not only will the wrong muscles be asked to support the body through the movement, the chances of injury will also increase.

Most of all, correct AFP keeps your spine healthy throughout your life. The spine is the most important component for function, but because it's so sensitive it must be protected at all times. If AFP is so poor that it breaks through the protective mechanisms of your body and allows your spinal cord to be damaged, this can result in lifelong pain and movement dysfunction. Damage the spine, and you will likely feel the effects for the rest of your life.

There are cultures of people living in third-world countries who can walk several miles with heavy buckets of water balanced on the top of their heads. Thanks to proper AFP, these individuals go through their entire life without the chronic back problems that are so common in western sedentary lifestyles. Our bodies are well-equipped to handle significant external forces—even balancing heavy buckets of water on our heads—if we maintain proper AFP. Lose AFP and a simple task like standing up can leave you injured for weeks.

There are no shortcuts and rewards for exerting yourself with exercise if it's at the expense of AFP. The greater and more frequent the deviations from AFP, the more likely you are to injure yourself. Never sacrifice AFP and ensure that the exercises you do are done with proper alignment, form and posture. If in doubt, ask a trainer to point you in the right direction.

…

No discussion about posture, form and alignment is complete without mentioning functional training. The reality of the situation is simple. We live in a modern world that demands ever-increasing amounts of time and energy to get by. Chances are that this pattern isn't going to end anytime soon, either. Movement and exercise strategies need to be time-efficient and effective in order to accommodate busy schedules. Attempting to train each muscle group in isolation, like biceps curls, would mean spending excessive time exercising. By training the whole body in one hit, you significantly cut down the amount of time spent exercising without sacrificing quality.

But there is more to functional training than just time-efficiency. Functional training prepares the body for everyday life, making daily tasks easier—and seemingly effortless—as a result. A functional training methodology acknowledges that your body is not a series of unrelated and disconnected muscle groups, but rather a single interconnected and complex organism. Every movement requires the whole muscular system to be activated and work synergistically as a single unit.[24] If your car breaks down and you have to push it, there's no luxury of sitting down to support your legs and core as you push, like you do with traditional machines in the weights room. Instead, the whole body must work as a single unit to perform the task. Forget training single muscles like the chest, biceps or quads. Train the entire organism so that it better translates to function required in everyday life.

When you go to the gym, focus on compound movements such as squats or lunges instead of single-joint movements like the leg extension or leg curl machines, and pull-ups or push-ups instead of biceps curls or triceps extensions. They replicate daily movement requirements more effectively, require more coordination and burn more calories based on metabolic demands over time.[25] They are simply more functional.

So train functionally. Choose exercises that move your whole body and challenge your strength, flexibility and coordination. Ditch the machines and move your body as a single unit. You get bonus points if you do it outdoors.

Healthy Habits: Movement

Movement and exercise strategies look different for everyone. People have different fitness levels. Some are more advanced than others and can effectively perform physically demanding tasks, while others lack motor skills and need to start with easier exercises. We all have different goals, too. Depending on an individual's fitness, performance and aesthetic goals, different movement and exercise strategies need to be emphasized. For example, someone wanting to get into body building is better suited to resistance training than yoga, while a competitive runner should definitely prioritize running. But despite the many variables that make your movement strategies unique, implementing and developing the following healthy habits will help you stay active your entire life.

1. Daily Movement

There is no single medicine or drug on this planet that will have the same degree of disease prevention and life longevity as daily movement. Scientifically speaking, daily and consistent movement is referred to as 'light-intensity lifestyle activities' and has been shown to improve all biomarkers for metabolic and cardiovascular diseases.[26] But you can call it 'walking' for short.

Walking is clearly a lost art. Hippocrates said that walking is man's best medicine, yet these days we're more likely to jump in the car and drive up the road to the supermarket or take the elevator instead of the stairs. For even a tiny investment of 15 minutes four times a week, walking is a surefire contributor to longevity.[27] Walking gets better and better for you the longer you do it too, with increased daily walking being linked to better health and longevity.[28] Simply put, the more you walk, the longer you live. And if you space your light-intensity lifestyle activities throughout the day, you actually reap the same benefits as one big long walk.[29] Make it your goal to take periodic breaks throughout your day to enjoy a brisk walk.

Make daily movement a habit by finding and creating opportunities in your everyday life to walk to and from destinations. When you drive to work, park a five-minute walk away from it. When you go to the store, park in the furthest corner of the parking lot. Take the stairs. Set an alarm to stretch every hour at work. Find ways to make movement a normal part of your everyday life because it's your best form of preventative medicine.

2. Exercise Intensification

The human body is an incredible machine. (Yes, even your body.) Most people don't know or understand their own physical capabilities because they've never pushed themselves hard enough. But the truth is that the body has an uncanny ability of adapting to the stresses that are placed upon it. If you want to be stronger, you need to consistently push yourself beyond your current limits. Your body will adapt. And when it does, you'll reap the physical and mental benefits that come with that adaptation. Over time, this skill will continue to improve and your strength will continue to increase. If you want be more flexible, stretch just beyond your capacity each time you do it. Your body adapts. It has to. This process is dictated by fundamental laws. Your body will adapt to the forces you place on it. The only thing that's required from your end is mindful and consistent intensification—and discipline.

Start jogging and running instead of walking to produce greater weight loss effects.[30] Increase the amount of time you exercise or increase the resistance you use during weight training sessions. Attend fitness or yoga classes that are above your current fitness level. The benefits you gain from intensifying your exercise are numerous.

Push yourself beyond your comfort zone to directly improve your health and longevity. In fact, combining low-intensity daily movement strategies like walking with vigorous and intense exercise is optimal for weight management and prevention of cardiovascular deaths.[31] It's important to note, though, that this doesn't necessarily mean to intensify your exercise to the point of physical exhaustion or fatigue; even seemingly small methods of intensification are good for you. Something as simple as increasing walking speed has been shown to substantially decrease mortality.[32,33] The resulting improvement in cardiorespiratory fitness—how your circulatory, respiratory and muscular systems supply oxygen to the rest of your body—associated with exercise intensification also helps prevent death caused by cardiovascular disease, despite often being overlooked in clinical environments.[34] High-intensity training has also been associated with greater fat- and weight-loss.[35,36,37]

Exercise intensification makes everyday life easier. If you push yourself during training sessions, playing with your kids or surviving a long day at work will be much easier. As you get older, you'll retain your independence for longer. More importantly, thanks to a lifetime of rigorous exercise, you'll also have the capacity to prevent falls and minimize injuries from accidents with a musculoskeletal frame that has been trained to withstand the random accidents of life.

Lastly, exercise also plays a role in the body composition and aesthetics. The general shape of your body is determined by the quality of your diet. If you eat a healthy diet consisting predominantly of Real Food, the shape of your body will be lean. Your movement and exercise strategy, however, determines the finer details of that shape. Consider how you exercise to be your personal Photoshop software program that controls, to a certain extent, which muscles are more pronounced, defined, larger or leaner. Exercise intensification plays a huge role here. It's really pretty simple; if you want the body of a sprinter, you need to train like a sprinter. Understanding how these athletes—or any athlete for that matter—train will help determine how, when and why you should intensify various parts of your exercise strategy.

The logic is simple: push yourself within the controlled environments of your workout so that you're better prepared for the uncontrollable variables and unforeseen randomness that life sometimes throws at you.

3. Diversify Movement & Exercise

Every type of movement and exercise—and more importantly *how* you maintain correct form, alignment and posture—provides different physiological benefits for the human body. Some improve flexibility and mobility, some improve muscular strength or hypertrophy, some improve your agility, speed and power, and still others improve your cardiovascular and respiratory systems. If your goal is health and longevity, you need all of them. Just like eating a wide variety of different foods is optimal for nutritional health, diversifying movement and exercise provides the best benefits for overall musculoskeletal health.

Balance is the goal. Anytime your body gets too out of balance, injury risks increase. Some weight lifters are able to bench press enormous amounts of weight but lack the flexibility to cross their arms in front of their body. Some throwing athletes and golfers rotate solely to a single side, causing structural imbalances that leave them prone to injury in their everyday life. Flexibility and mobility are important for optimal joint range of motion, but being hyper-mobile or hyper-flexible can increase the risk of injury.[38] Running can also be an excellent form of exercise with many health benefits, but solely relying on running as your only movement and exercise strategy increases injury risk.[39] Injuries that occur as a result of single-focused movement and exercise—as is often the case with recreational runners—illustrate the concept called pattern overload or overuse.

When an individual, irrespective of age or activity, engages in the same activity repetitively, connective tissue damage occurs where the repetitive strain is placed.[40,41] Because you keep performing the same activity over and over again, the tissues involved in the movement are never given time to adapt and recover, thus leading to tissue breakdown and overuse injury. It's no surprise, then, that the majority of injuries evaluated in running injury clinics are related to overuse, considering that running produces significant forces on many of the joints and muscles of the body.[42,43] If you run with poor form or alignment, these forces quickly lead down the inflammation path towards chronic injury. This is a prime example of pattern overload and overuse.

It's important to objectively assess your movement and exercise strengths and limitations in order to understand how to mix up your movement strategies. A hyper-mobile yogi may choose to incorporate strength training. Recreational runners can incorporate swimming or yoga to avoid some of the injuries associated with repetitive running while still benefiting from the cardiovascular and endurance aspects running provides.

Diversifying movement also results in neurological and metabolic benefits. By improving kinesthetic coordination, your brain stays fit, healthy and capable of continued learning too.[44] Plus, since your brain hasn't adapted to new movement requirements yet, you'll also need more energy to perform the task as your brain and body gets used to it, in turn also assisting with weight loss and weight management goals.[45,46]

Your body is an amazing adapter to the stresses you place on it. Make it a habit to periodically diversify movement strategies. Try it all: yoga, Pilates, resistance training, swimming, hiking or racquetball. Diversify your movement and exercise strategies to balance and enhance your movement qualities, help prevent injuries, train your brain—and have more fun.

Rest & Relaxation

"One of the symptoms of an approaching nervous breakdown is the belief that one's work is terribly important." – Bertrand Russell

"The mark of a successful man is one that has spent an entire day on the bank of a river without feeling guilty about it." – Author Unknown

Armed with a customized exercise and nutrition plan, David made incredible progress with his new healthy lifestyle. He lost weight, his clothes felt looser, he liked what he saw in the mirror, he enjoyed deep sleep through the night, and he found he had plenty of energy leftover after work to exercise. Life was good.

Then just as quickly as his enthusiasm buoyed, his progress came to a grinding halt. David had hit a plateau. He'd heard it happens to everyone so he wasn't that worried; in fact, he'd been expecting to plateau so he'd figured out in advance how he was going to tackle it head-on.

Despite increasing demands and longer hours at work adding a lot of stress to his life, David began exercising more and eating less. It was a strategy that seemed logical enough. Exercise more, eat less, lose weight—it's simple mathematics! To his surprise, though, the results were minimal, if at all existent. It turns out the human body doesn't pay much attention to simple equations.

So David decided to take it up a notch. He increased his exercise and lowered his food intake even further. The results? Nothing. No weight loss, no improvements in body composition and, worst of all, no energy.

David had assumed his 'exercise more, eat less' strategy was a foolproof and guaranteed way to bust through his plateau. Instead, it had totally backfired, and nearly every part of his daily life suffered as a result. His mental focus drifted. The quality of the work he produced at work declined. He had less energy and found it hard to fall—and stay—asleep. Adding insult to injury were pesky aches and pains all over his body. It just didn't make sense.

David's situation isn't an exception; it's actually one of the most common traps people fall into when they embark on new health and wellness programs. They see immediate results just weeks after starting out—*woohoo!*—then the results slow down or stop altogether. Introducing: the infamous plateau.

The typical knee-jerk reaction to an unwanted plateau is to push yourself harder. And harder. And harder. You exercise longer and more intensely. You make food portions smaller or cut out meals altogether. You start to feel tired, worn out and irritable. You suffer in the name of getting healthier, yet your strategy is actually harming your health. Without a continuation of the immediate results you experienced when you first started out, you feel like your efforts are in vain. So you push the envelope even further. Still no results. This pattern usually continues until you crash. You get sick, injured or depressed—sometimes all three. You've stressed your body too much and it's literally shutting down. Welcome to the world of overtraining. The only way out is to understand stress and how it impacts your physiology.

Stress: Pollution of the Human Ecosystem

It's time to revisit fifth grade. You're sitting in your seat and your teacher (let's call her Mrs. Smith) has just instructed everyone to put everything away except for a single piece of paper and pencil. That's right, it's time for a pop quiz. As your palms get sweaty and you nervously hold your breath, Mrs. Smith calmly walks over to the chalkboard and writes a single statement. *Name the oceans of the world.* You sit in your chair, eyes closed, imagining a map in front of you as you try to remember the world's oceans.

So, did you remember all five? If you did, pat yourself on the back—you did learn something at school! The Pacific, Atlantic, Arctic, Indian and Southern oceans span the entire geographic landscape of Planet Earth. Knowing all five might give you school credit, however the names of the oceans are merely labels that help with communication. They provide people with a basis for comparison and understanding. When you're talking about which beach you visited during your European vacation, knowing which ocean it backs onto creates a mutual understanding about exactly where you stayed, without having to open up an atlas. Strictly speaking, though, dividing and labeling the world's oceans is a mental construct that misrepresents the true nature of our world's ocean waters.

The reality is that the world's oceans are a single body of water. While waves sometimes mark where two bodies of water meet, like at the very top of New Zealand where the Pacific Ocean and the Tasman Sea meet, there are no real dividers marking the end of one ocean and the beginning of another. This single mass of water is also very intimately connected. In 2010 when 50 million barrels of toxic oil poured into the Gulf of Mexico after BP's infamous oil spill, the effects invariably impacted neighboring ecosystems and eventually the rest of the world's waters and networks. Traveling through the food chain and via oceanic currents, the toxic pollutants of the BP oil spill had global environmental impacts. Plant, animal and human lives all over the world felt the ill effects of this tragic event. That's because nothing happens in isolation.

In much the same way, the human body exists as a single entity too. Sure, we label different muscles, organs and systems to increase our understanding and improve communication, but they're really just labels. Substantively our bodies are single frames of connected and integrated parts, all of which inescapably impact one another. Our bodies have physical, emotional, mental and spiritual components that are made up of muscular, skeletal, visceral, fascial, neurological, limbic and hormonal systems, all of which are intimately connected. Just like the ocean, polluting any one of these systems will impact the body's entire ecosystem.

When you injure your lower back, the consequences reach beyond the obvious connective tissue damage. Anti-inflammatory hormones are released to initiate the healing process. Pain receptors and neurological pathways send signals to the brain when potential for pain is perceived. The surrounding lumbar muscles stiffen to protect the hurt part of your lower back. The combination of stress hormones and pain adversely impacts your mental and emotional states. You feel crummy, depressed and sour; you even take it out on others. Your entire human system is ultimately affected by a seemingly isolated lower back injury.

The human body is made up of systems within systems within systems within systems, all of which are fundamentally connected. The only significant difference between the ocean's ecosystem and the human body's interconnected systems is the destructive substance creating the pollution. While the Gulf of Mexico was polluted by millions of barrels of oil and chemical dispersants, our bodies are polluted with stress. A lot of stress.

Any experience that requires your body to expend energy is stress. And that's pretty much everything. Eating is a stress. Every bite of food that enters your mouth forces your body to utilize resources to extract nutrients and digest food, thus consuming energy. If your food is heavily processed, your body must work that much harder to extract and digest what it needs.

Breathing is a stress. When your body inhales air that's contaminated with pollutants, it must work hard to detoxify itself. Even clean air requires the body to burn energy in an effort to circulate the beneficial aspects of air throughout the entire body.

You've probably heard 'experts' recommend living a less stressful life to improve your overall state of mind, but if pretty much every single thing you do creates some kind of stress on your body, how is that possible? Well, the only sure-fire way to avoid stress altogether is to avoid birth. What this proves is that stress is actually a normal part of life, and a part that you're never going to escape from 100 percent. Our bodies are well equipped to handle most, if not all, of the stresses thrown in its direction. The question is how quickly they can recover.

The human body is a great adapter to stress. It takes stress from any source and directed towards any system, then distributes it all over the body in order to lower the direct effect it has on a single part of the body. The Godfather of stress research and science, Dr. Hans Selye, dedicated his life to understanding how stress impacts the body and how it responds to it. During his experiments on rats, Selye found that an organism would respond to any source of external biological stress by going through a series of steps involving the entire body to help restore balance. This is your interconnected human ocean. Your body simply adapts to the stresses placed on it in the only way it knows how: sharing the stress load with the whole system. It's a remarkable survival mechanism.

This is why you can throw a lifetime of bad habits and lifestyles at your body, yet it continues to function. Think about the poor lifestyle choices you've made. When we look at all the junk food we eat, exercise habits we lack, stressful jobs we keep and emotionally-draining relationships we participate in, it's amazing we still function despite the huge amounts of stress we place on our bodies.

Short-term periods of stress enhance human function, and in many ways are vital to survival. Acute stress fires up your adrenaline when you duck out of the way of an oncoming car after thoughtlessly stepping into the street, or when extreme sport enthusiasts jump out of airplanes or race down dirt tracks. Short-term stress even boosts mental capabilities to cope with the short-term demands and pressures of a mentally-challenging project. Acute stresses like these are beneficial in small doses. They're the good kind of stresses. You experience it, adapt to it, recover from it, then move on. The kind of stress you need to worry about is the unabated free flow of stress leaking into your body for long periods of time. Long-term exposure to stress can destroy your body's ecosystem.

Before the BP accident, the Gulf of Mexico's ecosystem had dealt with pollutants and toxins on a daily basis. The low level of severity allowed the Gulf to manage the pollution with naturally occurring currents that dispersed the insignificant amounts of toxins. The ecosystem stayed within an acceptable range of homeostasis—or balance—and any disruptions were quickly and efficiently managed. It wasn't until the overwhelming amount of oil stressed the Gulf's ecosystem that the system was thrown out of balance, creating significant environmental consequences all over the world.

This same phenomenon is true for the human body. It's not until the body is overwhelmed with stress from various sources and over long periods of time that it begins to malfunction. This is the world of chronic stress.

Chronic stress is like driving your car with the gas pedal all the way down. The engine pumps on all cylinders and the RPMs redline. Gas burns quickly. The tires screech and leave skid marks on the tarmac. The car races along the road.

Your car is designed to handle all that stress for a short period of time. The key phrase here is 'short period of time.' Your car is not designed to be pushed to the limit for long periods of time. It needs time to recover, time for the engine and tires to cool down, a chance to refuel and check the oil. Eventually, if you keep driving your car this way, something will break. In the same way, if you continue to live a stressed-out life, something in your body will break down or stop working altogether.

Today's non-stop, fast-paced world makes us live with constant and continuous stress. We drive on all cylinders without understanding that our bodies just can't perform at peak conditions forever. We work long hours at stressful jobs we hate. We spend our time with people who emotionally harm us rather than support us. We eat fast food and reach for sugary snacks throughout the day, stressing and inflaming our digestive system. We struggle to survive the working week so we can relax over the weekend, except our weekend recreation activities involve more stress like drinking booze and staying out late. No one should feel surprised when they get sick if they lead a life like this.

You start out healthy with all the capabilities of managing life's stresses. As your stress load increases without corresponding strategies for recovery, though, you become unhealthy. It's a dynamic process that ebbs and flows with every decision you make. If you consistently make choices that add unwarranted chronic stress to your body's ecosystem, your health will ultimately suffer. Like a collapse of dominoes, when one system begins to falter it stresses the other systems, leading to dysfunction. Stress—and the resulting inflammation—is at the root of nearly every human illness, especially the ones of the chronic variety.

Are you the type who reaches straight for junk food when you're stressed out? Stressed people eat more, usually of the highly processed and sugary variety. This is commonly known as emotional eating—and it's a real thing. Scientists have found that stress directly increases appetite; these cravings aren't necessarily linked to the body's lack of nutrients at a given time, but rather by stress being experienced.[1]

Stressed people exercise less, mostly because they don't have time for exercise—or because they feel like they just can't face it. Stressed people are constantly tired, yet they can't relax enough to get a good night's sleep. Stressed people have an altered immune function, making them more likely to get—and stay—sick.[2] Stressed people also have more heart attacks, more depression, more colds—and less sex. Chronic stress is at the root of all these problems. When you constantly run on all cylinders, it's not a matter of if but when your body will break down. You need to periodically take your foot of the gas and allow your engines to slow down. Periodic recovery sessions will ensure your body lasts the entire race.

Relax to Restore

As much as we dislike it, the irony of the situation is that stress is essential for growth. If you want to build muscle and lose fat, your body needs stress in the form of exercise. If you want to be an entrepreneur or run a Fortune 500 company, you better believe that stress will become an inherent part of your existence. If you want to be the best version of yourself and maximize your potential, overcoming stressful situations will be a normal and necessary part of daily life. But while stepping outside of your physical, mental and emotional comfort zones into stressful opportunities are necessary, stress is only half of the equation for progress and productivity. If stress is on one side of the seesaw, adaptation is on the other.

Your life's seesaw must be balanced. It's imperative to provide your mind and body with opportunities to adapt and recover from the many stresses placed on it. When you work out intensely, it's in the recovery period that your muscles grow, fat burns and all the other physiological benefits occur, not during the workout. The workout is just another stress—albeit a good one—that must be managed and adapted to appropriately. When you're working long hours—days or even weeks on end—stepping away from your work environment to rejuvenate is the most productive thing you can do for yourself and the company in the long haul. It's in the recovery process where all the magic happens. Even small investments in relaxing and restorative strategies will improve your health and wellbeing across your entire physiology.

Stress actually makes it difficult for someone to analyze and detect appropriate behavior for a given social situation.[3] That's why you often say things you don't really mean when you're stressed and arguing with someone. In contrast, the relaxation response releases muscle tension, lowers blood pressure and slows the heart and breath rates. When you're really stressed, relaxation techniques can provide you with the valuable time you need to take a step back and rationally assess a situation so you don't react emotionally and impulsively. These are sometimes the decisions that can have drastic consequences on your life, so it's better to approach them with an even keel and level head.

Relaxation techniques provide clarity of thought that allow for more rational decision-making overall, not just social interactions.[4] One study found that when stressed, people weighed risk and reward for decisions differently. Somewhat counter-intuitively, people tended to focus more on the positive and downplayed the negative aspects of a decision. This explains why people who are under significant stress in their job or relationship focus on the upsides of alternatives to their situation, rather than objectively viewing their circumstances and making a rational decision that also acknowledges the negative qualities of their decision. Have you ever jumped the gun on a decision simply because you felt extremely stressed in the moment, only to realize it may have been impulsive? Your mental landscape is like a snow globe. When significantly stressed, that snow globe is shaken and it's impossible to see clearly through the snow. Relaxation techniques allow the snow of your mental snow globe to settle so you can clearly see the situation and make appropriate decisions.

Restorative practices are nothing new. Many originated in traditional Eastern religions and philosophies, have been practiced for thousands of years, and are considered by some as essential components of a healthy and happy life. But one aspect of restorative practice that's always been a hot-topic among members of different scientific circles, is whether these restorative techniques can actually be approved by Western scientific studies utilizing new-age technology, rather than solely relying on what some called 'pseudo-science'. That's why a group from Harvard Medical sought out to quantify the physiological outcomes of mind-body interventions. This study focused on high-stress individuals who were prescribed restorative activities such as meditation and yoga, while scientists used neuro-imaging and genomics technology to assess the impacts of these various relaxation techniques on genes and brain activity.

Up until this point, countless studies had confirmed the mental health benefits of restorative techniques like yoga and meditation, but these studies relied almost entirely on the subjective experience and personal testimony of the participant, leaving very little hard evidence to be considered for skeptics demanding quantifiable and measureable data. The skeptics argued that if these restorative practices were beneficial to human health, they should create results that are measurable and comparable. That's why this study drew so much attention, because the technology utilized finally allowed biological effects to be tracked and measured.

Not surprisingly, the study confirmed what's been known for several hundreds of years by followers and practitioners of Eastern philosophies: mind-body interventions and practices influence the genes that control stress levels and immune function. [5] Whether the individual was new to these restorative practices or a seasoned restorative veteran, genetic expression associated with energy metabolism, mitochondrial function, insulin secretion and telomere maintenance improved. Additionally, genetic expression linked to inflammatory responses and stress-related pathways was reduced. Also interestingly, the more an individual committed to their restorative practices, the more significant the physiological benefit they received. Long-term practitioners displayed greater results across all of the measureable genetic variables, illustrating that the more frequently you engage in restorative practices, the better off you will be.

The common bond linking all restorative practices like tai chi, breathing, meditation and yoga is the focus on the breath, calming the mind and consciously releasing the tension being held in your muscles. Aligning these three qualities brings a wide range of physiological benefits. [6] It really doesn't matter what you label your preferred restorative practice, what matters is that you cover off these three qualities while you perform it, since they're what makes your chosen practice restorative and rejuvenating to the mind, body and soul.

The importance of restorative practices simply cannot be overstated when it comes to health and longevity. Just ask the people who practice restorative activities and are lucky enough to age with grace and vitality. In 2014 Misao Okawa—the world's oldest person living at the time—celebrated her 116th birthday. She boiled her longevity recipe down to three simple ingredients: real food, sleep and relaxation.

Remember, just like any other lifestyle, it takes time to master relaxation techniques, but it's a skill that only gets better with time. It requires conscious and intentional action each and every time you attend to it. That's why they call it a practice. There's no competition or concrete goal. There's only you, your breath and the intention to calm the mind and body. So be patient with yourself as you would with a child whom you are teaching. In many ways, it's your inner child that you're trying to teach with these practices. So be still. Breathe. Let go. Relax. Restore.

Sleep: The King of Recovery

The Dalai Lama once said that sleep is the best form of meditation. This is why sleep deserves its own section. You've probably heard this before but it's still worth repeating because, as is the case with so many healthy lifestyles, common sense rarely ever translates into common practice. You need high-quality sleep for normal physiological function. In today's world of constant psychological stress and daily demands, we need sleep more than ever—yet it's sleep that's most likely to be neglected.

There's no shortage of scientific research showing the physiological benefits of sleep. The benefits are so broad and far-reaching that some doctors believe they should prescribe sleep rather than pills and potions to patients. Sleep has proven to be instrumental in the prevention and treatment of metabolic disorders, because sleep disturbances and circadian rhythm disruptions are closely linked to harmful metabolic conditions.[7] One study examined over 375,000 individuals and found that insufficient sleep contributed to obesity, type 2 diabetes, coronary heart disease, strokes, high blood pressure, asthma and arthritis.[8] But scientific studies like this rarely, if ever, convince individuals of the importance of prioritizing sleep in their own lives. If that were the case, the countless studies about the harmful effects of cigarettes would have instantly stopped smokers from smoking. It takes more than a catch-phrase from an expert to convince people to change their lifestyles. Chronic metabolic conditions only happen to other people, so why think too much about how it could affect me when I've got other things to worry about?

The short-term ramifications of sleep deprivation—specifically cognition, performance and emotions—illustrate the importance of prioritizing sleep into your schedule, even when you've got important work projects on the line. Sleep deprivation significantly damages high-level cognitive function like innovative thinking and creativity. Interestingly, this cognitive degradation remains even after alertness is restored with stimulants like caffeine.[9] So despite your best attempts to remain creative and focused with those extra couple cups of coffee, nothing beats a solid night of uninterrupted sleep.

Sleep deprivation also impacts relationships and interpersonal communications. When you're involved in important conversations with a spouse or loved one, communicating effectively and responsibly will make sure you don't say things you don't mean. But if you're sleep deprived, you may process and interpret emotional information inaccurately, creating some very serious consequences.[9]

But what does sleep specifically do to our physiology that makes it so important for health and function? What biochemical responses are actually initiated by sleep? It seems that the magic behind sleep's positive benefits focus around how sleep protects the brain. Two studies explain this slightly differently. The first study shows that even after just one night of sleep deprivation, blood molecules start to concentrate and clump together, resulting in losses in brain tissue.[10] So if you miss out on a night of sleep, the physical structure of your brain will actually change—and suffer. The second study, performed on mice, found that the space between brain cells may increase during sleep, allowing the brain to flush out toxins that build up during waking hours.[11] Researchers of this study were surprised by how little flow occurred in the brain during waking hours, which further suggested that the way brain cells behave differs drastically between conscious and unconscious states. The many mysteries of sleep and how these structural differences impact other aspects of health are unknown, but what we do know is that sleep is essential to keep the brain and body healthy.

Lastly, proper sleep complements and supports other healthy lifestyles, drastically boosting their health benefits. Quality sleep increases the benefits of exercise and healthy eating in their protection against cardiovascular disease.[12] The combination of traditional healthy lifestyle habits like eating right and working out regularly results in a 57% lower risk of cardiovascular disease and a 67% lower risk of fatal events. Add sufficient sleep to the equation, though, and the overall protective benefit is even greater, resulting in a 65% lower risk of cardiovascular disease and an 83% lower risk of fatal events. Not surprisingly, adding quality sleep to the entire lifestyle creates exponentially greater results than just a single lifestyle choice.

But sometimes getting a full eight hours of quality sleep just isn't possible. If the busyness of your lifestyle means you pretty much always miss out on a great night's sleep, maybe it's time to take a page out of a toddler's playbook and take regular naps. Daytime naps for kids are extremely important for their development. Missing even a single daily nap has been shown to increase anxiety and decrease cognitive function.[13] Fast forward to your life right now and the benefits are strikingly similar. A quick afternoon nap session boosts learning and memory abilities and could offset the loss of sleep hours during the night.[14] As it turns out, maybe an afternoon siesta isn't about laziness after all. In fact, it might be the best thing you can do for your productivity.

Balance Working 'Out' with Working 'In'

A huge proportion of the population doesn't exercise or make it to the gym regularly, and that's a huge problem. But once someone musters up the courage to enter the gym, buy a membership and embark on an exercise program, a problem on the other side of the spectrum occurs: the people—and there are many of them—who spend hours upon hours a day at the gym. These people think that since exercise is a good thing, they should do it a lot and reap even greater benefits. But the fact of the matter is that they're doing too much of a good thing. They begin experiencing joint pain, excessively sore muscles, mental exhaustion and decreased energy levels. With this constant go-go-go lifestyle, they end up burning the candle from both ends.

The goal of a health and wellness program is to ultimately live as long as you can and free from pain and chronic disease. At the end of the day, working out is still a stress on the body and it must be recognized this way. It can either support a life of longevity, or it can sap you of strength and energy, and in turn impair your immune system and make you more prone to illness. Frequency, volume and intensity of exercise must be calculated on an individual basis, including the total stress load they can handle every day.

The goal is to train, not drain. That's why working 'out' must be balanced with working 'in'. You have to relax to restore. It's not about exercising for the sake of being better at exercising; it's about understanding your entire daily lifestyle and balancing it out accordingly. This is the only way to make healthy lifestyles last well into the long-term. If you don't, you'll continue to perpetuate a vicious cycle at the expense of your body. Work, work, work, crash. Work, work, work, crash. And repeat.

But exercise is only one part of the lifestyle equation. Your entire lifestyle must be analyzed to understand where, when and how much restorative activity can be introduced into your daily life.

Consider Bill. He has a career that he enjoys and finds fulfillment within. He works roughly 40 hours a week. He has no relationship stress, no kids and no pressing financial concerns, and he makes it a point to travel at least four times during the year. If Bill wants to start an intense exercise routine to get into shape, his total stress load would allow for such a program because the rest of his daily lifestyle demands don't overly stress him out.

Now let's consider Sarah. She works 60 or more hours per week in a high-pressure job. She's a single mom of two kids—one is an emotional teenager—and she's always worried about whether she'll be able to pay her next mortgage payment. Most people would agree that Sarah's life is significantly more stressful than Bill's. If Sarah wants to start creating a healthy lifestyle, it would serve her well to focus on restorative practices rather than intense exercise simply because her body is already under so much other stress. In Sarah's case, it's better to substitute working 'out' with working 'in', to allow her body to adapt to her already high-stress lifestyle.

...

Every single one of us reacts to and deals with stress differently. Emotions, thoughts, opinions and perceptions make the human experience uniquely different for everyone. Based on our past experiences and how our sensory information is processed, our bodies react to every situation with different chemical releases. The more unresolved stress or emotional scarring that comes from an individual's past experiences, the greater the likelihood negative emotions like anxiety, insecurity, loneliness, grief and worry will impact them.

In other words, our present reality is distorted by our past experiences. How you perceive the current moment dictates whether you see a situation as a challenge or a threat. If you see it as a challenge, you will likely tackle it head-first and with a positive attitude. If you see it as a threat, you will look at it defensively and under a high level of stress. Stress is in the eye of the beholder.

If we always feel like we're being threatened without ever objectively looking at the situation, we will create habitual behavioral responses that constantly send us back into states of mental and emotional stress, even if the situation is really not worth stressing out about. Our stress response is simply the sum of our emotional reactions to stressful situations over the course of a lifetime.

Perceiving a situation as a challenge rather than a threat,

though, makes all the difference in terms of physiological response. In one study, psychology students and faculty were asked how they responded to common situations in their field, like taking an exam or preparing a presentation. While common, these situations produce very different responses and emotions in different people. After the study, participants were evaluated based on their emotional responses and coping strategies for the hypothetical situation they encountered. Participants who saw their situation as a challenge displayed more confident coping expectancies, lower perceptions of threat and higher positive emotion than those who saw the situation as a threat.[15]

Whether you look at a situation as a threat or a challenge has significant implications for balancing working 'out' and working 'in' strategies. If all of life's everyday projects and tasks are fun, meaningful and worthwhile, your body's physiological responses will create a positive cascade of hormones, chemicals and behavioral responses. If this is you, then you can certainly handle more working 'out' and reap the many benefits associated with movement and exercise.

If, on the other hand, you consider yourself a victim and completely paralyzed by your life situation—regardless of how it may look to an outsider—the stress response will dominate your body, cause immune system disruptions and hinder all metabolic functions. How you look at the stressful things that happen to you every day therefore impacts how you cope with them. As you begin lowering and managing stress, your honest assessment of your life situations may change and evolve too, transforming into positive coping behaviors.

Western culture is constantly on the go. Being busy, accomplishing goals and overwhelming our physical bodies wins us esteem and societal validation. Few people—if any—really value being still, relaxed and recovered. It's high time this changed, because the benefits that come with simply slowing down to allow your body to recover have been proven to be an essential part of a healthy life.

Healthy Habits: Rest & Relaxation

Make time to give your mind, body and spirit a chance to refuel. As counterintuitive as it may seem, taking time to relax and decompress is the best way to maintain progress with a health and wellness program, not to mention improve personal and workplace productivity. With all of the energy that's created as a result, you can keep your new lifestyle journey going without crashing along the way due to over-work, over-exhaustion or over-stress. Learn how to balance the stresses in your life with appropriate and complementary times for restoration. Remember, it's a seesaw with stress on one end and adaptation on the other. Both are necessary, but modern lifestyles frequently neglect rest and relaxation. It's during recovery periods that all the magic happens. Look at fat loss and muscle growth: it happens outside of workout time, not during. Not sure where to start? These healthy habits will help you cultivate some much needed R & R.

1. Create a Sleep Routine

Like the other important tasks in your daily life, sleep must be scheduled. If it doesn't get added to the list of things to do, it'll simply be forgotten. The steps leading up to sleep are imperative because humans are creatures of habit, so the more we condition our body to know that it's time to sleep, the faster we'll drift off into high quality sleep. It's similar to Pavlov's dogs responding to bells by salivating in anticipation of being fed. If you develop a series of consistent behaviors and actions before going to sleep every night, then your body will start to understand that it's time for bed, and physiologically and biochemically respond in ways that will make it easy to wind down then fall asleep.

Obviously, there are good and not so good pre-sleep activities. Choosing stimulating tasks like watching TV or performing intense workouts aren't the best choices for a sleep routine. Instead, choose activities that are calming and relaxing. Turn off the TV and disconnect from your computer because the stimulation and light from television and electronic screens actually keeps you awake.

Take 30 minutes before you typically go to bed to read a book, meditate, stretch or listen to calming music—or a combination of all of them. Go one step further and plan the next day so it's off your mind. Whatever you decide is the best routine to get you in the mood to sleep, though, make sure you do it consistently.

2. Muscle Maintenance

It's true that our muscles need a challenge, but they also need a break. We hold tension in our muscles and connective tissue for a variety of reasons. Sitting causes unnecessary tension in different parts of the body. Mental and emotional stresses create neuromuscular holding patterns in the body that result in tight and achy muscles. Even working out can create tight muscles since consistent exercise breaks down the tiny fibers of the muscle tissue, creating an inflammatory response commonly recognized as soreness. When soreness is not managed appropriately, though, the tissues become chronically tight and limit range of motion and flexibility. This is why you sometimes see bodybuilders walking around the gym looking very stiff. When you neglect muscle tissue recovery for a long time, the tension increases to create extreme muscle stiffness.

Over time, any of the above examples can lead to pain and discomfort because tense muscle tissue misses out on good blood and oxygen flow. These tight areas of muscle, often called trigger points, can be painful to touch or even create pain in distant parts of the body when stimulated. The science behind trigger points is still in its infancy (plus we're still not entirely sure what a trigger point actually is) but what we do know is that caring and maintaining the muscle tissue is an important part of a restorative strategy. Just like our mental and emotional states, our physical bodies need pampering and stress reducing techniques.

When you book a massage, dedicate a big chunk of time to flexibility and mobility exercises, or perform self-massage techniques with a foam roller or tennis ball, you free up tight areas of the body that need more circulation, and open up range of motion in other parts of the body. As you remove tightness, you improve the general circulation of your body. Massage immediately after exercise also reduces inflammation and helps in the recovery process.[16]

Taking care of your body through effective bodywork alleviates anxiety, depression, tension headaches, digestive disorders, stress and pain, and improves soft tissue injury management, immune function (most likely from the improved circulation throughout your body) and sleep.

It's important to care for and nurture your physical body as regularly as you do your mental and emotional body. You only get one body; it's not like a car where you can trade it in for a new model when the old one refuses to start three days running. Aches and pains should not be ignored. Listen to your body because these minor physical discomforts could progressively evolve into chronic and debilitating injuries that significantly affect normal human function. Attend to your pesky muscle and joint pains with muscle maintenance techniques that fix the underlying problem, not pills and potions that just mask the symptom.

Schedule a massage twice a month, buy a foam roller and perform self-massage techniques yourself a couple times a week, or simply use a tennis ball to go after the tight areas. Just remember to care for your muscle tissue periodically to maintain optimal function.

3. The Art of Doing Nothing

Doing nothing may sound simple, but it's anything but. The moment you sit still, your mind begins to wander and you start fidgeting. Your brain starts thinking about all the things you should be doing that you aren't.

Don't succumb to the temptations; stay strong and sit still. When you do nothing correctly, you allow your body to recharge its energy reserves. The more common name for this practice is meditation. The true benefits of meditation occur because the body and mind are allowed—albeit forcibly at times—to be still and do nothing, resulting in much needed recharging.

There are three major forms of meditation. The first and most popular form of meditation focuses on an object or process like your breath or keeping your mind clear, rather than allowing the free flow of thought. The second reinforces change in one's environment by repeating a mantra over and over again, in order to create a desired outcome in a thought process or state. The third kind of meditation occurs when an individual reflects on good thoughts or things that have happened in his or her life. This expression of gratitude allows free flowing of thoughts as it goes from one positive thought to the next.

It doesn't matter how long you sit and meditate. Even if it's only for five minutes upon waking or before drifting off to sleep, meditation greatly impacts your mental function. It's like clearing your mind's cache or allowing a snow globe to settle after shaking it vigorously. Set your alarm at work or sit in meditation when you feel most stressed out. These five minutes will do more for your productivity, state of mind and stress relief than anything else.

4. Simplify. Simplify. Simplify.

The more you have, the more you stress—that's why many of the greatest thinkers in human history have endorsed simplicity. Enjoy the simple pleasures of life and get rid of the unnecessary. In order to bring new things in your life, you need to let go of the old first. Purge, toss and throw away the unnecessary junk in your life that only requires time and energy to manage. This could be anything. Throw away old and useless clothes. Clean and organize your inbox. Clean your house. Your physical space is sacred; keep it organized. The worst way to spend your time is managing things and stuff. The nature of things and stuff is that they get old quickly and require a lot of time, money and energy to manage and maintain.

It's easy to find happiness when you take a simpler approach to life. You'll be happier when you assess the quality of your day by whether or not you had a healthy meal, exercise and quality sleep. By focusing on the simple things your body needs for health rather than the short-term gratification of consumerism and materialism, you focus on what it means to be authentically human. Keep it simple.

5. Have Fun

In a world of constant deadlines and never ending responsibilities, it's important to regularly disconnect and just have fun. If you're worried that you won't get anything done if you have too much fun, consider that in times of relaxing fun some of the greatest ideas and solutions arise.

World champion chess player and Tai Chi champion Josh Waitzkin said that while other chess prodigies were practicing 12 hours a day, he would regularly take his boat out to sea and get lost in the beauty of the ocean. Can you guess what would happen during these regular outings? Waitzkin says he had his greatest 'ah-ha' moments about chess strategy. With his mind clear, complex chess problems would simply unravel. The most difficult chess questions seemed to answer themselves in these relaxed times away from the board. This same methodology can be applied to every project, career or job. Sometimes the greatest advances are made away from the frontlines, when the subconscious mind is free to roam for answers. Though it may seem like an accidental stumbling-upon, it's actually the farthest thing from the truth. These moments of clarity are the direct result of letting the brain rest, relax and integrate new information into its enormous database of connections.

Life was meant for fun, not work. If the latter was the case, we'd all be slaves to our circumstances. We have the power to choose what we do and how we do it. If we bring a sense of fun to our daily grind, at least we'll enjoy the long hours of work. It's only the constant and incessant cultural programming we're surrounded by that states otherwise. Having fun is stress-reducing and more productive than beating your head against a brick wall trying to figure out a solution. Having fun restores energy levels, heals the body and improves cognitive function. Having fun is simply good for your health and wellbeing.[17] Make sure to schedule regular fun events into your daily life.

Lifelong Learning

"Intellectual growth should commence at birth and cease only at death."
– Albert Einstein

"We now accept the fact that learning is a lifelong process of keeping abreast of change. And the most pressing task is to teach people how to learn."
– Peter Drucker

David's mother would be so proud; he's now eating better than he ever has, although he still likes to indulge in a few guilty pleasures every now and again. One night David's watching TV when out of nowhere a sugary craving kicks in. He wanders over to the pantry and opens it wide, his eyes hungrily searching for something that'll satisfy his hunger. Colorful cereal boxes complete with cartoon mascots on the sides neatly line one of the shelves. Just as he reaches for one of the boxes, he stops. For the first time, a little voice in the back of his head pops up:

Hey David, why are you reaching for the same cereal you've been eating since you were five years old? Didn't you just watch a commercial with this breakfast cereal character in it? Have you been eating this stuff since infancy simply because your TV told you to?

David chuckles to himself and closes the pantry door. He strides over to his TV, switches it off and grabs a book to read instead. In what seems like an epiphany, David resolves to no longer let television dominate his private life. In a deep moment of reflection David begins questioning just how many of his life decisions are determined by his television.

...

When discussing how lifelong learning impacts your health, we need to start with the flickering box that sits in the corner of your bedroom. The power of television in determining social behaviors is far more powerful than people care to admit. That's because most people—probably including you—believe they're not influenced by mainstream media advertisers and brands. Well, there's got to be a reason why companies pay more than $4 million for 30 seconds of airtime during the Super Bowl, right? Unfortunately, these people fail to recognize the extent to which television impacts subconscious behaviors.

Advertising companies and brands know the true power they possess. They have the ability to train and condition viewers into buying behaviors that will resonate so deeply that they stick with them for the rest of their lives. That's why David still eats breakfast cereals (complete with colorful marshmallows and cartoon mascots) whose cardboard boxes arguably have more nutritional value than the cereals themselves. The immaturity of young children increases their susceptibility to persuasive commercials for foods of poor nutritional quality too. Children request these unhealthful food choices while watching television and shopping.[1] This wouldn't be an issue if the advertised food products were actually healthy. Unfortunately, over 95% of the food and beverage ads on children's television programming are unhealthy.[2] Television is simply not appropriate for the development of adolescent minds. Children who do not have a limit on their daily TV watching time are twice as likely to drink sugary drinks every day.[3] More TV viewing is also associated with unhealthy eating habits that contribute to obesity.[4] But worse still is that advertising companies know and understand this very well. They employ the best psychologists and marketers in order to create lifelong customers for their junk that pretends to be food.

Since your subconscious mind was formed very early in childhood, it makes economic sense for advertisers to target this young and impressionable market. Your subconscious mind dominates the majority of your daily decision-making. It's a wise long-term investment for advertisers' brands and products, but it also means that we've been conditioned—brainwashed even—to covet brands and products that trigger emotional responses through their advertising. Not convinced? Look at the number of people who get injured or die each year in the middle of Black Friday shopping frenzies. It's sheer lunacy.

Most of the consumerism and materialism running rampant today is not natural. In fact, it's a product of the culture propagated by mainstream media. It's not until you turn off your TV and start interacting with the real world that you start truly learning. So ask yourself, what are you doing with your free time? The more we watch TV, the less we learn. Television tells us what to think, how to think, and essentially programs our behaviors with its content. To be a lifelong learner, you have to learn *how* to think. That inevitably begins when you start to think for yourself.

Schooling vs. Learning

I've never let my schooling interfere with my education. Mark Twain's famous words sum up the issues being faced by the public education system today. You'd be forgiven for thinking that going to school and receiving an education are the same thing. Unfortunately, that's not always the case. Of course it's not impossible to receive an education from your schooling experience, but just attending school, completing assignments and passing exams certainly doesn't guarantee an education.

Why? The fundamental reason why going to school doesn't automatically equal receiving an education is because in today's industrialized school model, students are taught *what* to think, not *how* to think. The former provides you with the skills you need to survive in the world, while the latter gives you the tools you need to thrive. If you want to become the master and commander of your own life, then you have to learn *how* to think.

Public education now closely resembles a factory in which a student is taken through set curricula and standardized tests, and comes out the other end a direct replica of the student sitting beside him. Memorizing facts and understanding how to beat tests are more important than creative problem solving and analytical skills. As result, we're judged by scores, grades and rankings. Earning an A+ on an assignment might make you feel great about yourself, but what's neglected in the traditional education process is a student's individuality including creativity, personal interest, culture, skill set, life goals and type of intelligence. Different people learn well in different environments.[5] To use the same measuring stick for everyone is a disservice for the entire system. Albert Einstein, one of the greatest—if not the greatest—minds in human history was right when he said that *everybody is a genius. But if you judge a fish by its ability to climb a tree, it will live its whole life believing that it is stupid.*

In one of his thought-provoking and entertaining presentations,[6] Sir Ken Robinson—one of the leading advocates for reforming public education—discusses current issues in education and how the static nature of our industrialized educational systems just can't keep up with our rapidly changing social environment. Without educational reform, Robinson argues that America's public education system will remain one of the worst in the world.[7] The one-size-fits-all model may work for car manufacturing, but it fails at education, thwarting individual creativity and diversity of thought in the process. Something is definitely missing from the public education equation.

The result has been increasing numbers of young adults questioning the necessity of public education and choosing to follow the path of self-education (some in lieu of and others in addition to the traditional model), and rightfully so since graduating with a bachelor's degree or beyond no longer guarantees the same career success it once did. Michael Ellsberg—author of *The Education of Millionaires*—discusses in his book how students nowadays are not taught how to survive and thrive in the real world because academic institutions don't cultivate the 'street smarts' necessary to do so. Instead of teaching valuable lessons such as finding meaningful and passionate work, finding great mentors, creating and making a vision a reality, money management, and marketing and branding yourself, schools teach prepackaged outdated courses that after third grade are rarely applicable to daily life.

The duty of public education should be preparing individuals for the demands of the real world, not for success on tests based on theory, which are often static and out of date due to the incredibly slow pace at which academic information can change or evolve. Instead, students across the country are now graduating with student loans the size of mortgages with nothing to show for it except a minimum wage job—if they're lucky. Both Ken Robinson and Michael Ellsberg agree that the traditional public education model does a really good job at one thing: training more college professors. Those who succeed are most often those with street smarts, not book smarts. Practical know-how trumps bottled industrialized academic theory. Just ask people like Mark Zuckerberg, Ralph Lauren or Bill Gates.

If you've spent significant time with young children, you know how imaginative and creative their thoughts are. Kids can leave you in awe and with the biggest smile when their creative thoughts surface. This is no accident because young children are right-brain hemisphere dominant in their early years of life.[8] Right-brain qualities like emotional expression, spatial awareness and creativity overshadow left-brain skills such as writing, logic and mathematics. It's a combination of parental, societal and cultural influences that pulls that beautiful and infinite imagination back down to earth, instead of nurturing and supporting creative expression.

The truth is, though, that society needs both left-brain and right-brain skills. This is the formula that produces better problem solvers, promotes open-mindedness and allows for acceptance of diverse thinking. Currently, though, the socioeconomic landscape is dominated by left-brain thinking and infrastructure. The few right-brain individuals brave enough to stand out have been the notable figures who have changed and revolutionized the world around us in enormous ways. Names like Elon Musk and Steve Jobs come to mind. Surviving in the real world today requires not only a firm understanding of logical facts and knowledge, but also the ability to apply that knowledge to emerging problems in creative and innovative ways. Break the industrial mold and don't allow schooling to interfere with your education.

Teaching an Old Dog New Tricks

As a culture, we have painted the aging process in the worst possible light. Physically speaking, aging is characterized by wrinkles, gray hair and failing hearing. Mentally, aging supposedly brings senility and declined cognitive function. No one wants to get old so we fight tooth and nail against it, even if only superficially with cosmetic surgery and the like. What people fail to realize, though, is that the process of aging is firmly in your control. The more you take care of your health now, the better you feel as you get older. Of course there's no way to escape aging, but it is possible to age healthily, and nowhere is that more apparent than with your mental capabilities.

Lifelong learning is a choice. There is nothing that prevents a person from learning new skills and engaging in new activities other than a lack of mindset or motivation. The problem is people get comfortable, feel scared or experience a combination of the two. Once those two emotions take over the psyche, every excuse in the book will be used to avoid educational opportunities that place people outside of their comfort zones.

That's why lifelong learning requires immense amounts of vulnerability and adaptability. It's hard to be a beginner at new activities, especially the older you get. It's even more difficult to question your core beliefs and have the courage to search for more knowledge—especially if you risk shattering your most fundamental beliefs. But the journey of lifelong learning is worth it. You'll begin to question authorities because finding the truth yourself is more gratifying and fulfilling than blindly following what someone else told you. And if you end up reaching the same destination as when you started, it'll be infinitely more valuable to you because you got there yourself, plus you'll be wiser for it. You'll put yourself in other people's shoes to understand their situations and perspectives, improving your own knowledge and growing in the process.

Keep in mind, though, that you do have to be comfortable with being wrong sometimes—because it will happen plenty of times.

In fact, being wrong isn't a negative at all; it actually helps you grow supremely more than being right all the time. Success and progress isn't measured by how many times you've failed. Rather, it is a measurement of how many times you choose to get back up and continue onward. Perseverance and resilience are the real measures of a successful life.

You may have heard the old saying, *you can't teach an old dog new tricks*. Well, that's ridiculous. Of course you can. And when you do, those new skills will keep your aging brain sharp and astute.[9] It's never too late to change. You choose how your brain—and your life—develops. You can redefine yourself by questioning your core beliefs and digging deeper. You could watch mind-numbing reality TV, or you could read self-improvement books. Each has drastically different outcomes on your brain.

If the process of lifelong learning—and thus *how* to think—had to be boiled down into a few simple guidelines, they would be as follows:

- Remain open-minded to as much input as possible.
- Don't shut out the feedback loop with personal judgment, prejudices and preconceived ideas.
- Objectively examine other people's points of view as if they were your own.
- Be self-sufficient and take responsibility for everything that happens in your life.
- Creatively assess any and all possibilities for a solution.
- Be willing to redefine yourself daily.
- Maintain the ability to take a step back and see the bigger picture, because there are always more variables to consider.

These guidelines establish the difference between knowing

what to think and knowing *how* to think. When you truly start thinking for yourself, you'll truly start learning rather than memorizing.

Healthy Habits: Lifelong Learning

Learning doesn't stop when school ends. In fact, for many people this is when real learning truly begins. The world is a constantly changing place and if you want to grow and develop alongside it, you must cultivate a hunger for learning, take the initiative and make the commitment to constantly expand your mind. You'll develop new skills or hone current ones, excel at being a conversationalist who can spark up discussions in any environment, and arm yourself with an intellectual compass allowing you to navigate through the world with grace and ease. Lifelong learning is a journey. Once you begin your quest, you probably won't stop. The more you know, the more you'll want to know. It's an insatiable thirst, but quench it responsibly. Enjoy the adventure with these healthy habits for lifelong learning.

1. Continued Education

The common theme throughout this chapter is that the more you learn, the more slowly, gracefully and healthily you will age. The secret to keeping your mental edge as you grow older is simple: commit to learning new things and refining current skills.[10] But *how* you learn—with regards to your mindset, intent and focus— plays a critical role in how much benefit you will gain.

They say that to become a master of a skill or expert in a field, it takes 10,000 hours of experience. While this number may or may not reflect reality 100% of the time, this simple explanation fails to take into consideration the level of concentration required of the practitioner. It doesn't matter how many hours you spend doing something; if you do it mindlessly and without heart-felt passion, it's a waste of time. Whatever activity you choose to do, whether you wish to become an expert in it or not, do it with an attitude of mindfulness and intention. Be in the moment and let the experience flow. Be there with all of your physical, mental and emotional presence. Do. Think. Feel. Combine the three for the deepest learning experience possible. You'll learn more and have greater cognitive benefits as a result.[11] The more you allow yourself to sink into the new experience, the deeper you will grasp the concepts.

Continued education opportunities are countless in today's modern world, plus they're easier—and cheaper—to access than ever before. Take courses at a local college or online. Try new outdoor activities that get you involved with groups or movements that are fun and exciting. Take up a new hobby or learn a new language. The world is truly your oyster. All you have to do is show up with passion, commitment and enthusiasm.

2. Read Daily

How many times have you been disappointed by the movie rendition of a great book? That's because movie studio technology can never fully capture, encapsulate and package the sheer power of your imagination. When you read a book that sucks you into its world, the movie that runs through your mind's eye is more vivid than any movie could possibly create. Sure, technology is getting us closer and impressing us with each new advancement, but nothing quite compares to the authentic experience elicited by your favorite books.

The power of reading is so much more than just entertainment, though. After a long stressful day of work, reading has been proven to be the ultimate relaxation, calming and restorative sleep preparation strategy—even more so than music, having a cup of tea or going for a walk.[12] Regularly consuming literary content keeps the brain sharp and cognitively acute, and helps stave off mental decline, an important factor in preventing Alzheimer's disease.[13] Reading has also been shown to have substantive clinical benefits to those who suffer from depression.[14,15]

By far the most important benefits associated with reading are the improvements in interpersonal communication skills. Reading exposes you to new ideas and deeper understandings of complex and broad subject matter. Reading provides you with shortcuts to gaining experience through the lives and words of other people. The perspective you gain makes you a more empathetic communicator who understands the mental states of others and the complexities of social relationships.[16,17] If self-improvement and personal growth are important to you, the development of these communication skills will be paramount to your long-term success.

Pick up a professional development book in your field of interest to expand your industry knowledge. Find a self-help book that addresses one of your weak areas as a form of personal growth. Escape into some fictional fantasy world after a long day of work. It really doesn't matter what you read; what matters is that you habitually make it a point to read every day.

3. Television Detox

Sedentary lifestyles are unhealthy—there's no questioning that. But utilizing that sedentary time to watch television is a special kind of unhealthy. For some reason, sitting on your sofa to watch TV is worse for your health than sitting in your car to drive to work.[18] A lot worse.[19] Even playing video games and completing computer work are associated with less harmful effects, despite both being sedentary activities.[20] At least with video games, you required to use finger-eye coordination as well as critical thinking skills, depending on the game. Similar to playing violent video games, however, watching television is associated with anti-social and aggressive behaviors.[21] The circumstances surrounding this issue are still largely unclear, but mounting evidence continues to highlight television's adverse impacts on human health, even if you only have it on for background noise.[22] When you consider that television is largely a marketing tool for companies with budgets large enough to get their products and services on your screen, you can see why the whole equation is flawed. TV is not for your benefit.

In developing countries where technology is still relatively new—and rare—television ownership is associated with a massive 400% increased likelihood of obesity, 250% increase in diabetes, 31% decrease in physical activity and 21% increase in sitting when compared to those who don't have television.[23] All in all, television is responsible for significant tolls on the quality—and quantity—of your life. Every hour of watching TV shortens your life by an astonishing 21.8 minutes, making TV viewing time comparable to major chronic disease risk factors such as physical inactivity.[24]

Given that the educational value of most television content is nil, is it any surprise that this mindless activity is so bad for your health? The reality TV shows that dominant the landscapes of network television provide substantively nothing to viewers other than opportunities to be sold commercial brands and products. It's time to put down the remote control and detox from television— even for just a short time. And if you truly can't sum up the courage to unplug from your daily fixes of favorite sitcoms and programs, do yourself a favor and get it out of your bedroom. That action alone can impact your sleep quality,[25] your sex life and, more importantly, your waistline.[26]

Television—the physical product itself—does not cause these health problems directly. It's not like a television carries some kind of contagious disease that, once caught, wreaks havoc on human physiological systems. The main concern with television is that it displaces time that would otherwise be available for healthy activities. Instead of watching TV, fill your schedule with activities that are beneficial for your health and add substance to your life, such as exercise, reading, socializing or hiking. There really are an infinite number of options. If you get confused or overloaded with options, a good place to start is one of the many habits available in this book.

4. Travel Somewhere New

Traveling is not only an incredible learning experience; it's also the height of human experience. Anyone who disagrees has yet to join the exclusive fraternity. Travelers are among the friendliest bunch in the world who enjoy sharing the pleasure of life's simple moments in the company of other like-minded travelers.

So why is traveling the foundation of just about every person's bucket list? What is it that makes the experience of travel so relishing? Why do people slave away, working long hours at work, only to thoughtlessly spend life savings—or max out credit cards—buying one-way tickets? It's quite simple, actually. Traveling is the epitome of living in the moment. Time somehow slows down. To travel is to live mindfully.

Traveling inherently means stepping outside of your comfort zone where thinking on your feet is the name of the game. Your everyday routines are broken and the autopilot switch turns off. A mindless commute to work transforms into a jigsaw puzzle of opportunity. Even if you're the kind of person who plans everything down to a tee, traveling forces you to problem solve and live completely in the moment. This kind of unfamiliarity breeds innovative and creative response. You can't rely on the programmed behavioral patterns that work so well for you in the office; instead you need to rely on instincts, street smarts and a sprinkle of common sense. The confidence and adaptability gained while traveling will equip you for anything life throws your way. If you can handle traveling, you can handle anything.

Living in a single location for an entire lifetime is like reading a single page out of a book. By traveling, you open yourself up to an endless supply of stories. The best part is that you'll become a storyteller for the rest of your life. Traveling instigates authentic and deep relationships with people, immerses you in new cultures, and excites your taste buds with local cuisine. If nothing else, you'll gain invaluable knowledge and worthwhile perspective. Your deeper understanding of the world will make you more easy-going, relaxed and accepting of the world—and people—around you. That's why Mark Twain famously said that *travel is fatal to prejudice, bigotry and narrow-mindedness, and many of our people need it sorely on these accounts.*

Traveling is good for your health and should not be postponed until retirement or old age.[27] Your physical, mental and emotional wellbeing will improve when you pack your bags and journey off to somewhere new.[28] In fact, traveling can play a significant role in the prevention of chronic disease.[29] We already know we're not guaranteed anything in this world except for the present moment. Live for today. There is no better way to taste life's experiences than through travel.

Traveling doesn't necessarily require visiting a new country or state, either. Neighboring cities have plenty of new things to try that maybe you never realized existed. Even if it's just across town or finding a completely unique way of commuting home, discover and explore the world around you and soak it all in. Be creative and have fun. Educational adventures await.

Community

"Healing is impossible in loneliness; it is the opposite of loneliness. Conviviality is healing. To be healed we must come with all the other creatures to the feast of Creation." – Wendell Berry

"You are a product of your environment. So choose the environment that will best develop you toward your objective. Analyze your life in terms of its environment. Are the things around you helping you toward success - or are they holding you back?" – W. Clement Stone

David has completed another week of healthy eating habits, daily exercising and relaxation strategies, and he feels pretty good about it. The weekend arrives so, like clockwork, he heads off to hang out with his friends for their usual Friday night festivities featuring a lot of eating, drinking and being merry. Now that David's focused on healthy living, though, he doesn't really enjoy nights of eating fast food and drinking until he passes out anymore. His friends' hearts are definitely in the right place so the peer pressure they place on David isn't intentional or coming from a negative place, but they just don't get it. They behave and react like they always have done, but David's being dragged down with them.

After yet another weekend of mindless social eating and drinking, David immediately feels the difference in his health—physically, mentally and emotionally. He loves his friends and they love him back, but they simply don't know how to support his new healthy lifestyle. They don't see how important these new health goals really are to him. More than anything else, David wants to integrate his healthy lifestyles into his social circle so his friends can benefit from their own new healthy lifestyles. He suggests going hiking as a group instead of booking a Saturday afternoon table at a restaurant, but they jibe him at the sheer madness of the suggestion. He suggests hosting a healthy potluck where everyone cooks their own dish and they meet up at someone's house to share their creations, but his friends would rather order French fries and hot dogs than get creative in the kitchen. He attempts to start up a conversation about the benefits he's experiencing from meditation, but is greeted with raised eyebrows and silence. His friends just don't get it. They don't understand where David's coming from and are obviously firmly set in their comfortable—and unhealthy—ways.

Despite spending quality time with the people he loves, David always comes away from his weekends feeling … well, kind of lonely. It's hard for him to describe, because it's not like he has no friends, but as he heads in one direction towards better health and wellness, he feels more and more isolated from his friends. He used to have a lot in common with them; they've spent every weekend—and most weeknights—together for as long as he can remember. But now as he tries to transform his life for the better, he feels completely alone.

David heads to his parents' place for some much-needed love and support. His mom's love language is doing stuff for her family, so he can guarantee that seconds before he steps through the door she'll have put the kettle on for fresh coffee and set a steaming hot chocolate cake complete with jam and cream at the table ready to serve. She's the type who won't take no for an answer, so he doesn't want to offend her since he knows how important it is to her to do things for her family. David's father loves to relax in front of the TV. He subscribes to more cable channels David knew existed, and spends his hours watching history documentaries, movies and sports while his wife waits on him hand and foot. His dad suffers from type 2 diabetes so he stabs himself with insulin needles multiple times a day, yet he does very little to improve his health situation—and refuses to acknowledge the hard work he'll need to do to deal with it. Plus, the doctor said it's genetic and lifestyle changes supposedly won't make much of a difference anyway, so why bother? After a few hours of family time and more slices of chocolate cake than he cares to admit, David leaves with a feeling of guilt, regret and quite honestly sheer exhaustion after sitting around doing nothing but eating and watching mindless television programming all afternoon.

At work, the situation is much of the same. David's colleague, Martha, has been in the job much longer than he has, and her constant complaining about how much she hates her job and their boss is beginning to take its toll on his own sanity. David's started wearing headphones while he works to improve his concentration, but what Martha doesn't know is that there isn't actually any music playing, it's all just an illusion to make it look like David's very busy and doesn't want to be interrupted. David can't understand why Martha doesn't just leave and find another job. After all, she spends more time at her desk than she does at home, which means she's disillusioned with the majority of her life. That can't be healthy for anyone.

David sadly realizes that if he's going to continue tackling his health and wellness program with the same gusto and level of success he's seen so far, his future progress is at the mercy of his weakest link—his social network. The people he spends the most time with just don't share the same values, ideals and goals that he does now. He wants to continue learning about and discussing the many aspects of health and wellness, but the only conversation he can drum up is which bar will have the best happy hour specials, what's next on TV, or how awful his boss is. He's changed—and they haven't.

What makes matters worse is that David takes significant steps backwards every time he hangs out with his friends. He makes short-term sacrifices to satisfy the group and to avoid looking like an outcast. How can he truly expect his friends and family to understand his healthy ways? In comparison, they live unhealthy lives and complain about being overweight, always being tired, or being so overworked they just don't have time for anything else, yet they accept their circumstances as the norm, never questioning their own daily lifestyle choices. David starts to realize that the people he surrounds himself with play a significant role in his own health and wellbeing. How significant that role is, however, is greater than David could ever understand.

The Five People You Spend the Most Time With

It runs in the family. How many times have you heard that statement? While genetic and hereditary factors prove that there is a fair amount of truth to that statement, environmental factors also carry significant weight when determining the how and why of a person's health. Depending on the disease or condition, these environmental factors may play a stronger role than even genetics. This is especially true for chronic conditions, which have been shown to be lifestyle-oriented and thus preventable.[1] One chronic condition often blamed on genetics is obesity.

There's a funny cartoon circulating the internet depicting an obese patient talking with her doctor. In the cartoon, the doctor is looking at the patient's charts with the caption *the problem isn't that obesity runs in your family, the problem is that no one in your family runs.* While this over-simplification of the problem doesn't communicate the multivariable nature and complexity of obesity (it's the whole lifestyle that counts), it does raise an interesting question regarding the shared behaviors of family members. If you eat, move, laugh, work and, most importantly, think like your family members, it's likely that your health will bear a similar resemblance too. Here's where emerging science has stepped in to show us just how powerful our social networks truly are, family or otherwise. The results are quite astonishing.

One study evaluated a densely interconnected social network of more than 12,000 people from 1971 to 2003. The study found that a person's chance of becoming obese increased by 40% if their sibling also became obese during any interval of the study.[2] Some would argue that much of this increase in likelihood was due to genetic or hereditary factors, but the study also found a similar result when comparing normal friendships outside of family ties. If you were a participant in this study, your chances of becoming obese during this 32-year study would have been 57% more likely if one of your friends also became obese. This does not make obesity a contagious disease; rather, it proves the power of social networks and the behaviors they accept as normal.

When discussing obesity, it's just as important to examine non-biological lifestyle and behavioral factors as it is genetic and hereditary factors. As social creatures, we feed off each other for acceptable social behaviors. Another group of researchers out of Arizona State University concluded that you're more likely to adjust your dietary and exercise behaviors to meet the socially-accepted definitions of health and body image established by the group of people you spend the most time with.[3] In other words, if your friends eat well and work out regularly, you're more likely to also. In another meta-analysis, researchers found that if participants were told their friends were making low-calorie or high-calorie food choices, the likelihood that they too made similar food choices significantly increased, not to mention the amount of food they consumed.[4] This highlights the true power of the social network, and why Facebook has become such a large and successful company.

We look to our peers for lifestyle guidance, whether it be directly via verbal communication or indirectly by watching and listening. It's a classic case of monkey see, monkey do, and it reveals the importance of community-wide interventions when considering clinical and public health approaches to preventing obesity.

If the power of the social network can have such a massive impact on obesity, then it makes sense if that same impact could be measured on weight loss and health as well. And, as expected, this is precisely the case. Two studies looked into the role social networks play when applied to weight loss challenges and adopting heart-healthy lifestyles. The first study showed that weight loss was clearly clustered within teams, illustrating that teammates influenced each other's behaviors.[5] The second study was aimed at promoting and implementing heart-healthy lifestyles, and the results were again consistent with the expectations of the social network phenomenon. Behaviors and lifestyle choices are contagious amongst the people you spend the most time with. In this case, people in support social networks together lost an average of 6.5lbs more weight, trimmed an extra 1¼ inches from their waists, and had 4 to 5 mmHg drops in systolic and diastolic blood pressure readings.[6] What we can conclude from studies like these is that individuals within social groups will, more often than not, share many of the same values, goals and expectations. That is, after all, why they choose to be in a group together. The people within these social groups have exponentially more accountability and motivation for their goals because they have the backing and support of the likeminded community.

As you can see, community-accepted social norms impact individual behaviors on a very significant level. This makes the people you spend the most time with a very important part of your life. These people can truly make or break your goals. If they're supportive, motivating and like-minded, they can help you get to where you want to be faster and more effectively. If they're on a totally different page, they could stop your progress altogether. As the old saying goes, *you are the average of the five people you spend the most time with*. If you analyze the lifestyles, behaviors and habits of the closest members of your social network, you can paint a realistic picture of who you are as a person, especially when it comes to what is and what isn't socially acceptable behavior. Chances are that there'll also be physical similarities in weight or body fat percentage since lifestyles have a direct impact on body composition.

If your goal is health and wellness, make sure the people closest to you will support your goals and lifestyle. This will create more opportunities for accountability, motivation and learning. Like-minded individuals keep each other accountable. Health-conscious individuals motivate each other. If the entire social group is inherently health-oriented, you'll educate and teach each other and dig deeper together as you learn more about health and your own body.

One is the Loneliest Number

We live in a time of supreme social connection. At least, that's what it looks like on the surface. We have multiple social media profiles that eat up much of our precious productivity time at work. Social media activities are so prevalent, in fact, that many employers now *expect* that significant chunks of an employee's day will be spent scrolling through their respective Facebook newsfeeds. We have web applications and smartphones that connect us with people on the other side of the world in seconds. You don't just hear your grandmother's voice on the other side of a telephone connection, you actually see her on your phone as if you were having a face-to-face conversation. We know these technologies are commonplace, widespread and mainstream *because* your grandmother can actually use it.

Yet, despite these technological advancements designed to improve the social connection between people, many of us still struggle with loneliness. That's because there's no substitute for authentic social connection—the kind you get from being around a real person. The sheer abundance and frequency of these superficial interactions via technology simply cannot replace authentic social connection, as much as companies and their technology platforms claim they can.

In modern day urban living, it's commonplace to live alone in an apartment or home. Because we're alone—yet evolved to be social creatures—we attempt to quench a fundamental human need with technological substitutes like texting, Facebook and online forums. Yet the more we try to engage and connect using these technologies, the lonelier we feel.[7] One study tracked how frequently participants interacted with Facebook, and found that increased usage and greater consumption of Facebook content was directly associated with poorer overall wellbeing and authentic social connection.[8] When it comes to social connection, there's just no substitute for the real thing.

As we attempt to live an individual-based lifestyle of self-actualization, self-realization and self-awareness, we find ourselves fundamentally lonely. Although these personal journeys of self-discovery are important for an individual's life satisfaction, there must be balance because it's actually within communities and social environments that we thrive. Frankly, loneliness is detrimental to health. Even if you're surrounded by friends, family and loved ones, the *perception* of loneliness will hinder immune function and increase the chances of heart conditions.[9,10,11] It's the mental and emotional feeling of loneliness that matters, not how it appears to be on the outside. Unfortunately, that feeling is more prevalent today than ever before.

As people grow older, community and social support becomes even more important for healthy aging and longevity. In fact, targeting emotional loneliness and social isolation could mean several more years of living for elderly people. Researchers from the University of Chicago studied more than 2,000 people aged 50 and over, and found that the loneliest participants increased their chances of premature death by 14%.[12] While social and emotional interventions like developing satisfying relationships played a critical role in helping those lonely individuals, improvements in physical health and wellbeing also helped reduce levels of loneliness. In other words, healthy eating and exercise habits can help prevent the perception of being socially isolated, alongside strategies that develop and maintain solid social relationships.

Nurturing and strengthening social bonds should not be held off until the last years of your life. Social engagement and participation will make you healthier and happier—now.[13] You need a social support system with people who will motivate and inspire you, regardless of your age. These are the people who will not only keep you motivated and focused on your short-term healthy living goals, they could literally be the lifeline that keeps you vital and energetic for the rest of your life. Healthy aging is almost always the result of strong community ties. Just ask the inhabitants of Blue Zones, small areas around the world where an unusually high percentage of inhabitants live to be 100 years old. These centenarians will tell you how important community support truly is.

Super Strength of Social Support

In the kidney-shaped mountainous Barbagia region of Sardinia, Italy, you can walk into a bar and find locals laughing and drinking together in what looks like a scene out of a movie. They curse, yell and argue. Shortly after, they grab a glass of wine, embrace one another, laugh it all off and rejoice with a resounding *Salute*—then start all over again. This culture of shepherds finds joy and satisfaction in the simple things in life. Their family unit is the most important thing to them and they often spend their entire lives living with multiple generations under one roof, thanks to a combination of both necessity and love. Mostly love.

Thousands of miles away, the celebrated and widely studied people of Okinawa embrace simplicity and moderation as a way of life. They eat slowly and strictly adhere to a calorie-restricted diet. They consciously refrain from binge eating, not for the sake of losing weight, but to allow themselves to listen to the infinite wisdom provided by their bodies with every bite of food they take. They regularly practice Hara Hachi Bu, the Confucian philosophy of eating until feeling 80% satiated. Their bodies tell them when they're satisfied, not empty plates. They enjoy diets high in vegetables and infuse their foods with herbs, seasonings and spices that provide as much health benefit as palate satisfaction. They regularly stop in the middle of their daily walks to bask in the glory of the sun, just to soak it all in. In times of economic hardship, the people of the Okinawa community band together and suffer bad times equally. When everyone bares the hardship, a single person does not feel it significantly. That's why the tightly-knit community of Okinawa has thrived for generations.

Even the United States has a unique Blue Zone culture in sunny California. The Seventh-Day Adventists of Loma Linda can generate enough positive energy in a single day to operate a city for a year. These fun-loving, outdoors-enjoying, adventurous folk don't stop moving until the day they are proudly taken from this existence. They treat family, friends, strangers and especially themselves in exactly the same manner: with abounding love. The strong community-wide spiritual practice dictates that they should not stress or worry about parts of their life they have no control over. As a result, they don't bother stressing out about the little things and instead focus their energies on other more important things—like having fun.

What all of these cultures have in common is their classification as a Blue Zone, regions discovered by Dan Buettner that are characterized by highly condensed regions of centenarians, or people who live past 100 years of age. Buettner's Blue Zones are scattered geographically across the globe. It makes sense, then, that their cultural ways of life differ substantially. These different cultures have to adapt to different climates, geographic settings, social landscapes and surrounding species of animals and plants. Different variables require different solutions.

The Okinawans eat slightly different diets than the Seventh-Day Adventists, who exercise and move differently than the Italians of Sardinia, who in turn have their own idea of what rest and relaxation entails. Each lifestyle is built on the variables surrounding each of their respective environments. The differences, however, are only superficial.

One of the most defining features of Blue Zone cultures is the profound respect for the elderly. Blue Zone inhabitants have an unspoken commitment that all members of society—particularly those who are most vulnerable—should be taken care of as well as possible. In every Blue Zone culture, not only is healthy aging the norm, but elders are honored, celebrated and revered. In America, seniors tend to live apart from their children and grandchildren, often sent off to retirement homes when they become unable to care for themselves. But that doesn't happen in Blue Zones. A combination of family duty, community pressure and genuine affection for elders keep centenarians with their families until death.

The sense of community and social support is greater within Blue Zones than anywhere else in the world.[14] Blue Zones put family first, keeping aging parents and grandparents nearby, and sometimes housing as many as four generations under a single roof. Not only does this build a social network that supports healthy behaviors, it provides vast amounts of wisdom and knowledge for younger generations as they learn to grow and survive in the world together. They always have someone to ask for help who truly has their best interests at heart, not quarterly profit margins and shareholder wealth.

This is not an argument for advocating moving into your parents' home and offering your grandparents the remaining spare bedroom—although the Blue Zones do prove that this could be beneficial for your health and longevity. What this does show us, though, is the importance of community and social support when developing healthy lifestyles. The stronger the community, the stronger the individual. Blue Zone cultures are the extreme representation of what that would look like since family bonds are lifelong bonds, both figuratively and physically.

We need social support to thrive. In fact, strong social ties keep us healthy by strengthening our immune systems and making us less likely to catch the common cold.[15] And if susceptibility to the common cold doesn't impress you, then consider that social support is also strongly associated with reductions to all-cause mortality risks. A meta-analysis reviewed 148 studies (more than 300,000 participants) and found that participants with stronger social relationships had a 50% increased likelihood of survival from all-cause mortality.[16] This finding remained consistent across age, sex, initial health status, cause of death and follow-up period. Researchers concluded that the influence of social relationships on risk for mortality is comparable with other well-established risk factors, such as lack of physical activity.

Living with several generations under a single roof like the inhabitants of Blue Zones may not be possible—or desirable—but the action provides real-world examples of what health and vitality can look like for elderly people when a support structure is available to them. Getting older doesn't necessarily mean getting sicker. It is possible to age gracefully and healthily with the help of a community that has the individual's best interests at heart.

The Community Within

Have you ever truly contemplated the epic vastness of the universe? Just look up at the night sky and gaze at the seemingly infinite number of shining and flickering stars. You can't help but feel awestruck—and, quite frankly, insignificant—after a few minutes of quiet stargazing. In order to restore your feeling of significance, however, all you have to do is move that steady and intentional gaze inward. Your body is literally a universe of its own. Trillions of other organisms call your gut, skin and other organs home. Indeed, foreign organisms actually outnumber your own cells 10 to one, and account for several pounds of your body weight.[17] Gross, right? Well, only if you don't understand how precious these organisms really are and how much you really need them for optimal health!

The truth is, what we classify broadly and generally as 'germs' co-evolved with humans over millions of years, which is also why the relationships we have with our foreign residents are, in many cases, beneficial for a wide variety of human functions such as digestion or cleaning skin. In fact, the relationship between you and your personal microbiome is very symbiotic. You need them just as much as they need you.

Attempts at living in a bubble to protect yourself from the world will ironically leave you defenseless. Children who grow up in sterile environments are more likely to suffer from asthma and allergies than children allowed to run around outside and get covered in mud every now and again. This is because your immune system requires germs, bacteria and foreign organisms to mature properly. As a child's developing immune system interacts with a wide diversity of foreign substances, it grows stronger and more capable of handling threats in the future. Much like how your muscles require stress to grow stronger and how your brain requires mental challenges to get smarter, your immune system needs to be exposed to the environment to become healthy and capable. Small exposures challenge the immune system. A minor cold, fever or infection is the perfect workout for your immune system. Rather than attempting to numb or rid your body of pesky symptoms like a cough or runny nose, sometimes letting your immune system handle the load naturally is a wise investment for the future. As the old adage goes, what doesn't kill you makes you stronger.

The foreign organisms that call your body home are—quite literally—your oldest friends. They've learned to live with you—

and you with them—for millions of years. Rather than being a fearful landlord and evicting your bacterial guests with sterile environments and overuse of antibiotics, learn to understand your natural bacteria and nurture your relationship with them. They're an intricate part of your body's complex universe. Indeed, fermented foods, pre- and pro-biotics, and the occasional rolling around in the dirt are far more likely to keep you healthy than excessive attempts at sterilization and extreme personal hygiene.

Healthy Habits: Community

Human beings are inherently social animals. One of the primary driving forces behind the evolutionary success of humans as a species was the ability to cooperate and forge strong social ties. Families and communities were respected and valued above individuals. What was good for the group was good for the individual. Times have changed, though, and strong communities are not as important for survival as they once were. Instead of seeking advice from our parents and grandparents, we ask Google. Today, we also get to choose our friends, spouses, families and communities, whereas in the past these were largely decisions made for us. In generations before us, broken commitments to the community could mean social ostracization. Today, we have no such binding commitments to communities or bonds. What remains constant, however, is that the people you choose to surround yourself with are important because they will greatly influence your behaviors and lifestyle—and therefore your health. These community-focused healthy habits will help with just that.

1. Find Your Cheering Squad
The people you surround yourself with help to dictate a significant portion of your health and wellbeing. Take a close look at your

social network and assess whether these people add to or subtract from your life. Let's not beat around the bush here; this is often a very difficult assessment to make, especially if some of the people you love the most like your family and long-term friends are the ones who aren't supporting you. However, in the long-term your ability—or inability—to do this important task can be the difference between the healthy life you desire and the chronic disease you fear the most. These are sometimes really tough decisions to make, but surrounding yourself with a cheering squad will be an important step in your health and wellness journey.

An effective cheering squad should be comprised of people who will make you more accountable. Their focus on their own health will motivate you to stay focused on yours. You'll discover new group activities that direct you towards your own goals. When you have a bad day or fall a little bit, they'll be there to help you back up again. These are the immovable rocks in your life that you can count on for support and motivation when you need it most. And because we're naturally competitive creatures, your cheering squad will provide some good healthy friendly competition as you push each other to improve in various aspects of your healthy lifestyles.

Find a local community group to join using resources like meetup.com. Host a potluck. Organize hikes. Just go and find your people. It may start with a single person, but it will grow if you continue to put yourself out there. These are the people who will help you become the healthiest version of yourself. They will be your rocks. They will help you succeed—and you them.

Of course this doesn't mean you should disown your family and life-long friends if they don't quite get where you're going with your new healthy lifestyle. It simply means that in order to keep moving forward with your health and wellness goals, you need to establish other relationships with people who are committed to mentoring, encouraging and leading you towards greatness. Yes, continue to hang out with your old friends when you can. Yes, keep heading along to weekly family dinners. But start looking to your new communities for the support you need to keep striding towards your goals, and learn to manage the amount of influence your family and old friends have over your new life. Maybe—hopefully—they'll learn to understand one day. Until then, you can't afford to let their opinions impact you in a negative way.

2. Cell Phone Detox

As a culture we've mastered and spent countless hours expanding our social media and the technical skills necessary for digital communications. All the while, though, we've neglected the neural pathways necessary for effectively communicating and interacting with actual people. We become proficient in what we practice most, and dealing with people face-to-face is just not one of those things. In fact, face-to-face interaction is such a foreign concept nowadays that university courses sometimes have to specialize in interpersonal communications.

Interpersonal skills—the ability to socially engage with other people—are the most important skills for life success. There's a reason why Dale Carnegie's book *How to Win Friends and Influence People* is still in print and referenced today, even though it was written in the 1930s. If you're not familiar with this book, don't be fooled by the title; it provides incredible insight and advice for dealing with other human beings, in person. How to communicate effectively and authentically listen to other people are just two of the gems inside the leaves of this book. The first and most crucial step in these social interactions is to actually be present. So get off your phone.

Let's face it; we all have a bad habit of staring at our phones at all hours of the day. We use them as alarm clocks, then spend 20 minutes before we get out of bed scrolling through the 'news'. They intrude on our social interactions. In fact, they stop social connection altogether. If you're going to be a part of a community, make sure you actually connect with the group by getting off your smart phone during social gatherings, events and outings. This can only serve as a foundation and formula for fulfilling friendships and opportunities you never thought possible, all made possible because you decided not to walk past people staring at a screen.

If you spend time with someone, leave your phone in your bag and engage in authentic human conversation. Pay close attention and actually listen to what they have to say. Listen more. Ask more questions and make it a point to learn something from every interaction you have. Your interactions with people will be more substantive, deeper and meaningful. You'll learn more. You'll feel better. More importantly, the person you're conversing with will feel better too. That's the greatest feeling of all: improving the mental state of the person you're hanging out with.

3. Reconnect with Nature

Get outdoors, enjoy the sunshine and get in touch with your primal roots. It's crazy that the outdoors are now more associated with an alternative 'hippy' lifestyle than normal life. Given that 99.999% of our history takes place in nature, our apartments and homes are actually the alternative. In fact, these dwellings have contributed to severing our intimate relationship with nature, where we've thrived for millions of years.

The sad reality is that some people are actually scared of the outdoors. That's a real shame since many aspects of nature have been proven to be beneficial for health. Aside from the well-documented vitamin D benefits associated with sunshine, exposure to sunlight has been associated with weight loss and BMI improvement, especially when exposure happens in the morning.[18] Exercising outdoors rather than indoors provides greater increases in energy and enjoyment, not to mention improved mental wellbeing.[19] In fact, spending time in nature has been shown to reduce stress and facilitate physiological relaxation as well.[20]

These benefits have been scientifically quantified and measured. Nature and outdoor advocate Yoshifumi Miyazaki and his team of researchers conducted experiments involving 420 subjects in 35 different forests throughout Japan. Spending time within natural surroundings resulted in 12.4% decreases in cortisol levels, systolic blood pressure and heart rate, plus improved immune function.[21] Miyazaki believes that nature therapy can and should play an important role in preventative medicine.

Nature deficit disorder is the popular theory that human beings—especially children—are spending less time outdoors, and their health is suffering as consequence. While nature deficit disorder has not been clinically recognized, over 40 studies have been compiled and reviewed and show not only the increasing absence of direct experience with the natural world, but also how this lack of experience impacts our health overall.[22] Disconnecting from nature has brought with it unintended consequences that impact our physical, social and emotional wellbeing.

So the moral of the story is: get outside and enjoy the many health benefits of our natural world. Go on nature hikes. Exercise outdoors. Reconnect with the natural community.

4. Practice Random Kindness
The mindset of community is truly practiced when you perform

acts for the benefit of others, with no expectation of gain for yourself. Albert Einstein famously said that you're here for the sake of helping others, and that your own wellbeing and happiness depends on it.

There's hardly a substitute for the fulfillment experienced after giving to someone or some cause. When you're busy helping and giving to others, you don't have time to stress about the trivial and monotonous stresses happening in your own life. There are real-problems in this world that deserve attention; the fact that your kids intruded on your only day to sleep in is not one of them. Helping others—especially those less fortunate than you—has the amazing ability of putting things into perspective and highlighting what really matters. When you look at the appreciation and gratitude you receive from the other side, it's no wonder many dedicate their lives to altruistic causes.

Not surprisingly, research shows that giving behavior is also tremendously healthy, with altruistic behaviors being associated with increased levels of happiness, lowered levels of depression, and positive results for those suffering from chronic diseases.[23] Kindness gives us healthier hearts, slows the aging process and makes us happier.[24] And like all social behaviors, kindness is contagious.[25] Start a domino effect and practice random acts of kindness. Do something or give something to someone who doesn't deserve it and can't give anything back, and enjoy the health benefits associated with selflessness. Practice random acts of kindness.

Love

"To love yourself right now, just as you are, is to give yourself heaven. Don't wait until you die. If you wait, you die now. If you love, you live now."
– Alan Cohen

"Stress is the distance between where your thoughts are and where your life is happening." – Dean Jackson

"Be here now." – Ram Dass

From the outside looking in, David now lives a very successful healthy lifestyle. It's taken him a lot of time, effort, discipline and dedication, and quite frankly, he almost gave up a few times, but he's pushed through and completely transformed his life. These days he eats a diet predominantly compromised of real food; movement and exercise have become as habitual as brushing his teeth; and he regularly schedules time off to rest, recover and recuperate from the stresses of everyday life. He loves hiking in the Great Outdoors with his new like-minded friends, but he also relishes the chance to get away from everything and everyone, and spend some quality time meditating and reflecting on life. He's even joined a local Toastmasters group for continued learning with a fun and supportive community.

From the outside, his life looks pretty sorted. From the inside, though, it's another story. Every day, away from the public eye, David fights cravings and temptations for self-destructive behaviors like drinking alcohol or eating sugary snack foods. When he isn't fighting these cravings, he's succumbing to them. When he gets stressed out at work, he reaches for candy. In the evening, a glass of wine helps David unwind. But when his emotions grow stronger and beyond a manageable level, cravings turn into all-out binge sessions or drunken nights. One square of chocolate becomes two blocks, plus a tub of ice cream. One sneaky glass of red wine becomes a few bottles with old friends. A hangover kicks him down for two days, then as he slowly regains control of his headache and bleary eyes, he feels like he has to start all over again. A deep sense of regret and self-loathing starts to creep in—but to look at him from the outside, no one else would ever realize the torment that goes on in his head.

This is the behavioral pattern David deals with pretty much every day of his life. In times of feeling inadequate, insecure or self-loathing, David numbs uncomfortable emotions like fear, anger and depression with unhealthy behaviors that provide short-term gratification and pleasure. Reaching for alcohol and sugary snacks is his escape. While they're only Band-Aid solutions to deeper problems, in the moment it just doesn't matter. David just wants to *feel* better. And this is how he's been programmed to cope with emotions his entire life. Feel bad. Consume. Numb the pain. Sweep it under the rug and deal with it later—if ever.

David needs to realize that these self-destructive behaviors stem from a deep-rooted lack of self-acceptance and self-love. But that's easier said than done. It takes a lot of courage to admit there's some serious stuff going on inside. In fact, few people have the courage to go deep within and learn about themselves in such a deep and intimate way. It requires a lot of emotional awareness and vulnerability. But the truth of the matter is that most of us—if not all of us—deal with the same human emotions every day of our lives. While our physical and mental worlds may be different, all humans substantively share similar underlying emotional currents, whether they're aware of it or not. Emotions are universal.

...

The final step of the healthy lifestyle puzzle is figuring out how to change the negative and self-destructive voices inside your head into positive and supportive ones. If you reconcile your negative emotional states and learn how to cope with uncomfortable emotions in constructive ways—not through self-destructive and numbing behaviors—you'll develop the tools necessary to make your healthy lifestyle a lifelong certainty. How? Well, the only way to make any healthy lifestyle sustainable is to disrupt and change the programmed behavioral patterns that have sabotaged every one of your past attempts at healthy living. This process begins and ends with love. Specifically, loving yourself.

Simply put, love is the glue that holds a healthy lifestyle together. Without it, a healthy lifestyle is one emotional breakdown or stressful situation away from falling apart at the seams. When you love and respect yourself, your ability to deal with uncomfortable emotional situations prevents you from falling back into destructive behavioral patterns—especially ones that involve poor eating choices.

We all know that eating healthy is important and we know what healthy food looks like, yet as soon as we feel uncomfortable, stressed, worried, even bored, we reach for unhealthy foods at a moment's notice. In times of discomfort, we use food as an escape. We know that dysfunctional relationships with careers, spouses or loved ones are harmful to our health, yet we continue to sacrifice our mental and emotional health by going back for more. We know drinking and smoking are destructive, yet we reach for them at the first sign of stress and discomfort. Rather than assess and address the emotion peeking its head over the horizon, we're conditioned to numb it with external substances like food, alcohol and even violent behaviors. We look outside to cope instead of inside to reconcile. In order to truly love ourselves, then, we need to go straight to the source: our emotions.

Your Emotional Beach Ball

Imagine trying to hold a fully-inflated beach ball underwater in a pool. It's hard! You have to carefully apply pressure across the entire surface of the ball, because it's constantly trying to fight its way to the surface. To fully submerge the ball is nearly impossible, unless the ball is mostly deflated. As soon as you lose focus or miscalculate the pressure, the ball shoots out of the water, splashing everyone around you. Everyone gets wet from the residual water of the explosion.

That's how our uncomfortable emotions work. We think we always need to keep our emotions hidden and subdued, but when we lose focus or become distracted, our emotional states erupt and splash everyone around us with their severity. We say things we don't mean and hurt people we never intended to. Everyone gets wet. Worse yet, that beach ball you're trying to control is inflated more and more every day with new emotions flooding in from the other things that happen to you on a daily basis. As the beach ball inflates, it gets harder and harder to control underwater.

Even if you don't mean it, everyone around us is impacted when our emotional beach ball shoots out of the water. Usually these situations and circumstances lead to conversations that start with *I don't know what came over me, I didn't mean what I said* or *I feel like I completely lost control*. Do any of these phrases sound familiar? The funny thing is, though, when you say those phrases you're probably being totally honest. It's *not* your conscious mind that vomited all those emotions on anyone unlucky enough to be around you. You didn't intend to hurt anyone. What happened, though, was a reaction from something in your subconscious being poked and prodded to the point of explosion. Your conscious and rational mind was overwritten by the much more powerful subconscious mind, which as it turns out, pretty much runs the decision-making show, whether you're aware of it or not.[1] Roughly 95% of our neurological processing abilities stem from our subconscious mind compared to our conscious mind; based on that massive statistic, which 'mind' do you think will win in the middle of an emotionally charged situation like an argument with a loved one?

The sheer complexity of the subconscious mind is well beyond the scope of this book, but how your subconscious mind relates to healthy lifestyle choices can be simplified and generalized as the following:

Your subconscious mind is comprised of the programming and behavioral patterns you learned in your first few years of life— many specialists agree on seven years—that help you cope with and manage the real world. These behavioral patterns are designed to protect you in the face of discomfort and attack, so when you have an emotional response and your beach ball threatens to thrust its way out of the water, your subconscious mind does all it can to keep it underwater, and keep you safe and healthy, based on the information it was programmed with during your childhood.[2]

Long before your emotional beach ball starts to create rifts in every aspect of your life, though, you use all of your conscious resources to manage life's situations without any emotional reaction at all. You learn to keep the beach ball in control by numbing and sedating the emotion with every bite of delicious food you eat. A bite of that delicious Ben and Jerry's ice cream pushes the beach ball down a little farther. A nice glass of Sauvignon Blanc makes everything all better. This strategy might work for a short while, but where did you learn it? And, more importantly, why were you taught to avoid these uncomfortable and negative emotions rather than acknowledge and deal with them? Therefore, do emotions play a key role in determining your lifestyle choices and consequently our likelihood of preventable chronic illnesses like obesity?

As it turns out, mental and emotional wellbeing may play a significant role in obesity, but we commonly overlook and disregard it since it deals directly with our childhood, our emotional experiences during childhood, and the strategies we learned back then to cope with our emotions. This has little or nothing at all to do with feeling 'good' or 'happy' all the time. In fact, this mindset is actually at the root of the problem. We constantly strive to feel good and happy rather than just *feel*. Other uncomfortable feelings—pain, fear, anger and depression—are deemed as socially unacceptable, so we learn to ignore them, to push them back under the water. As always, parents play a critical role.

Stressed out and insecure parents who lack practical methods of dealing with childhood emotions—most likely due to the inability to deal with their own emotions—react to their children's anger and sadness by consoling them with sugary snacks or additional TV time.[3] Similarly, children are often forced to finish their plates or are only allowed sugary dessert as a reward. These type of emotionally charged dietary behaviors play a significant role in the development of childhood eating behaviors because they alter the relationship between the child and their food, and instead turn food into a reward or some form of emotional soothing. Rather than a child feeling an uncomfortable emotion and the parent helping the child to understand and manage that unfamiliar or uncomfortable emotion, he or she is instead conditioned to sedate the emotion with lifestyle choices that significantly alter the mind-body relationship, and inhibit emotional reconciliation and growth. You can see why they call it emotional eating, and why it can quickly create a spiral of behaviors that lead to depression and obesity.[4]

From a young age, we're taught that our uncomfortable emotions aren't normal; that we shouldn't feel angry, sad or depressed; that we need to be happy and feel good about life all the time. We keep our negative emotions bottled up, so we feel bad when they unintentionally come to the surface. We begin to feel depressed about feeling depressed because we're taught that our emotions are unnatural and abnormal. It's a vicious cycle that stems from a society that places unrealistic expectations on people and values material success—achieved in any manner necessary—above all else.

Rather than using food as a coping mechanism for stressful situations, children suffering from low self-esteem, anxiety or other uncomfortable emotions need to be given early intervention strategies that improve their chances of long-term physical health. Children need to be encouraged to respond to their emotions, not numb them with dietary and lifestyle distractions. This type of short-term gratification and shortcut to parenting can have lifelong implications on behavioral patterns and unhealthy coping mechanisms. We're programmed to ignore uncomfortable emotions—they're bad and shouldn't exist. Somehow this is supposed to make the emotion go away. Of course, that simply doesn't happen.

As a parent, you have an enormous responsibility to your children to listen, acknowledge and accept their emotional states in the moment. Love them unconditionally, and encourage and guide them through every kind of emotion they display without judgment. These precious early moments of life will play the most significant role in their lives because a loving childhood has been shown to be one of the best predictors of mid to late-life health, happiness and success.[5] Fortunately the pressure doesn't just sit on the shoulders of parents. Culture, as a whole, plays an important role as well.

More than 5,000 teenagers across 19 countries were used in a study that indicated that young adults based their self-worth and self-esteem on whether they fulfilled the value priorities of others within their cultural environment.[6] Personal values seemed to have little or no influence on their self-regard. Individual self-esteem, then, remains consistent and in line with the values of our dominant culture, rather than personal values.

The dominating culture, then, has placed unrealistic expectations on the individual. The goals we're expected to make are unrealistically lofty, but failing to reach them is unacceptable. The only acceptable outcome is massive success, at any cost. As a result, we're often too hard on ourselves. One aspect of our culture is the notion that emotions like depression, anxiety, anger and sadness are inherently *bad*. We get depressed about being depressed. Then we medicate ourselves to numb a normal human emotion that has been inappropriately amplified, because our learned coping strategies are designed to discourage, hide and numb them. As we feel these unacceptable emotions and associate them with unacceptable states of being, our self-esteem suffers. We feel a bad emotion and subsequently numb that emotion with behaviors we feel bad about later. There's no escape from this feedback loop, and we only reinforce and solidify a behavioral pattern that destroys our self-esteem.

As a consequence, our self-esteem is damaged at an early age. We simply do not feel comfortable in our own skin because not only do we not know how to handle our emotional states, but we have not been provided with effective strategies to cope with such emotions—except to push the problem down the road to deal with later. But these poor coping mechanisms only turn into lifelong issues that impact your health as you get older. It's difficult to unlearn programmed responses, especially when we're not aware of them. And the self-perception you carry as a child impacts your health as an adult. Researchers assessed roughly 6,500 10-year-olds for emotional problems, self-perceptions and BMI. At the age of 30, the test subjects were again asked to report their BMI. The study found that those children with lower self-esteem at age 10 were more likely to be overweight 20 years later.[7] Therefore, unresolved childhood emotional patterns compounded by inappropriate coping mechanisms join forces to create an underlying psychological mindset with an inherently higher risk for obesity.

While mental and emotional stress may not be directly linked to obesity, the behavioral patterns and coping mechanisms created by inappropriately dealing with emotional stress through food consumption are. There's a reason why it's called comfort food. We know what healthy food looks like, yet we eat food that instantly gratifies our bodies and provides instant pleasure. It's a method for suppressing and coping with uncomfortable emotions. It's an escape from reality. This is why direct knowledge of what is healthy and what isn't is only part of the solution. The underlying behaviors driving the decision-making process are just as important.

Emotional eating does two things. First, it means you externally manage stressful situations with consumption behaviors, without actually dealing with the root cause of the problem. You program yourself to deal with emotion this way for the rest of your life. For some it could be food, but for others it could be excessive exercise, alcohol, sex or violence. Still others become workaholics in order to keep their beach ball from surfacing. A popular choice of emotional avoidance today is busying oneself on a smartphone. But the truth is that they're all working towards the common goal of numbing, avoiding, suppressing and ignoring uncomfortable emotional states. This is our programming, instilled in us as children, and it's sabotaging our efforts to sustain health lifestyles.

The second thing externalized coping behavior means is that we've never fully recognized, acknowledged and experienced the emotional states from our childhood. If we never reconcile these childhood emotions, they'll continue to torment us 10, 20, even 30 years down the track. As these emotions resurface in our lives, it gets harder and harder to suppress them, so the actions we take in the external world must match that intensity. That's why our coping behaviors usually become more intense as we get older. Some of us turn to harder and stronger drugs, while others' small acts of nastiness or bullying turn into horrific acts of violence. Our own uncomfortable emotional states are to blame, so we keep running from them. But the beach ball always finds a way to shoot out of the water, eventually.

Love is Now

It's pretty commonplace to worry about the past and fear for the future, but all the while the present moment passes us by. Rarely, if ever, is there attention—and direct intention—placed on the present moment and what's happening in the now. Right now. Instead, we waste our days by living in a fantasy world—one that has either already passed us by, or one that we can't really do anything about until it arrives.

The opposite of dealing with uncomfortable emotions with externalized coping behaviors is to let the present moment be what it is and appreciate it for what it really is. If you feel depressed, don't mask it and pretend it doesn't exist. *Acknowledge* it. *Feel* it. Don't feel bad about it. If you're angry, don't bottle it all up to deal with some other time—because that will probably end up being never. Tune into your body, try to experience that anger full on, and notice all the little ways your body reacts to that emotion. The same holds true for fear and every other socially stigmatized emotion in the book. Acknowledge the emotion and deal with it in the now.

This does not necessarily mean you need to act out on the negative emotions you feel—especially since your actions will always have consequences. You may feel angry, but acting out that anger is not the same as fully experiencing and feeling it. If you act out, you simply pass your anger onto someone else to feel and deal with. While this might make you feel better initially, remember that feeling better is not actually the goal. The goal is to feel the present moment as it is. The goal is to feel the anger and be okay with it. Like all other emotions in life, it will pass. And when it does, your beach ball will deflate a little bit at a time, making it easier—and less burdensome—to manage.

Authenticity is key here. If you're being asked to join in on an activity that you don't want to do—like a night out for drinks—just say no. If you're not coping with your workload at work, step into an office and talk to your boss about it; don't take on excessive amounts of work, letting the stress become more than you can handle. Learn to say 'no' when you mean 'no'. Don't compromise your personal integrity just to be nice and polite for sake of it. Be careful not to turn into a people pleaser when your underlying emotions are brimming to the point of overflowing and your helpful actions are inauthentic and forced, because shortly afterwards your beach ball is likely to thrust itself out of the water, splashing everyone around you in the process.

The path to present-moment appreciation is ultimately through truthfulness, honesty and genuineness—especially with yourself and your interactions with the world. Authenticity will set you free. The internal push/pull battles with yourself will disappear and you'll feel at ease when you're not constantly thinking one thing but doing another. You may upset a few people—or maybe even lose a few friends—with your honesty and directness at first, but at least you know the interaction was *real*. It was you. Don't be afraid to speak your truth. You're not trying to be perfect; you're being authentic. As you shed the inauthentic residues of the past, new opportunities present themselves that are in line with your authenticity.

What's different about this approach is what happens in your internal world. Instead of trying to shun the uncomfortable emotions and pretending they don't exist, acknowledge them and admit that they do exist. But also remain mindful not to project or act out towards others with your uncomfortable emotional states. Vomiting your emotional state onto others is not feeling it; it's just another form of escape. You have to *be* with your emotions. If you don't, they'll show up later in life—usually much stronger and more profound.

To make matters worse, you'll continue to attract people and life situations that trigger the same emotions that you've yet to fully experience and allow to pass through you. This phenomenon of reenacting and manifesting past emotional drama is known as the Creation and Manifestation of Reality theory in the world of psychotherapy.[8] Take a few moments and think about the many relationships and situations that you've taken part in that leave you saying *this always happens to me*. You may find that despite changes to your spouse, job or location, the same emotional states keep popping up over and over again. When you become fully aware of these reenactments, it's actually quite fascinating to watch it unfold. Some would call it entertaining. It's equally as amazing to know and appreciate that life provides you with seemingly endless opportunities to deal with and reconcile the emotions you've been running from for so long.

Love everything you feel when you feel it, because it's normal. Everyone feels uncomfortable and negative emotions. It's part of the human existence. It's life. But eating or drinking them away only makes the problem much worse in the long run. Be comfortable with discomfort. Love what's in the now. *That* is true and successful self-love. Experience it fully now, or allow it continue pestering you for the rest of your life.

We live in a society that's depressed about being depressed. In order to grow emotionally and bring reconciliation to our lives, we must be okay with the emotions that we feel, even when they're not always 'pleasant'. If we can learn to find love and beauty in the moment, we will become happier. Our tolerance of the world and people around us will grow. We'll start to communicate and interact with people authentically, rather than let our insecurities and suppressed emotions pollute every interaction and individual that may pose a threat to our preconceived and suppressed emotions.

It's okay to be angry, depressed, scared or anxious. Experience it fully. Tune in and really *feel* everything that is happening when those emotions turn up. You don't have to react. You have free will and can choose to use it, regardless of how emotionally charged a situation may feel. Viktor Frankl said that *between stimulus and response there is a space. In that space is our power to choose our response. In our response lies our growth and our freedom.* That space of time that Frankl is referring to is your opportunity to feel all the sensations associated with the present moment, and then—and only then—you can respond consciously and fully aware of the situation. In fact, most of the time it's better that you don't outwardly react at all to whatever's triggering the uncomfortable emotion. Just watch and tune in. It's your emotion to be felt and experienced, not anyone else's. This is your life. *Feel* it.

Conscious Reprogramming

How, then, do you reprogram your mind, feelings and actions, when ignoring them, bottling them up and moving on without dealing with them have been the norm since childhood? How do we start to deflate the underwater beach ball, even if it's just a little bit?

Let's cut to the chase: it's not an easy feat to change a lifetime of habit. It takes time—sometimes a lifetime—because the subconscious mind is like a mental recording playing on repeat. The subconscious mind produces knee-jerk reactions and feelings that seemingly come out of nowhere, yet they're just normal habitual programmed responses.

Here's one way to start to chip away at your habitual emotional responses. Exercise your power of free will and take action with your conscious mind. It's your conscious mind that gives you the choice to act in the moment and decide whether or not to listen to and act upon the knee-jerk subconscious reactions you feel. As hard as it may seem in the moment, you can overcome emotional urges with intentional practice. Use your conscious mind and conscious responses to impact your physiology by taking actionable and intentional steps towards self-love.

Even the smallest physical manipulations can impact your physiology and biochemistry. Here's an example. When someone is happy, they will smile. Millions of internal physiological responses stemming from the positive emotion will trigger a smile across a person's face. The funny thing is that it works in the other direction as well. Scientists have found that by simply holding your facial muscles in the shape of a smile, physiological and psychological benefits can occur during stressful situations.[9] So this means that you could feel better, even if you force a smile! And while this may seem like small potatoes at first glance, researchers have found that smiling is associated with slowing your heart rate, reducing stress and increasing overall happiness too. So fake it 'til you make it and make a smile happen, even if you don't feel it at all. You will eventually.

If the small muscles of the lips have this much power over physiology, imagine what you could do if you recruited your entire brain! The power that your conscious thoughts can have on your wellbeing is massive to say the least. For the sake of your health and vitality, it's important to shift your conscious mind's energy toward positive, life-generating thoughts, and eliminate energy draining and debilitating negative thoughts.

Positive thinking directly impacts your physiology and wellbeing. The more positively you think, the better it will be for you. Studies have shown that people with realistic or poor self-perceptions tend to be moderately depressed or suffer from low self-esteem, while overly positive people are much happier and healthier.[10,11] But positive thinking does more than just impact your individual health and physiology. One study aimed at disproving the hedonic treadmill, which is the concept that even though positive and negative events such as becoming paralyzed, winning the lottery and getting married can temporarily alter our levels of happiness, people quickly adapt to these states and return to their original emotions. If this theory were true, though, our attempts to improve happiness through methods such as positive thinking would be doomed for failure before starting. Instead, the participants in this study who implemented and regularly practiced positive thinking techniques such as loving kindness meditations, produced increases in daily experiences of positive emotions, especially when interacting with others.[12] The study also found that participants experienced increased mindfulness, sense of purpose, social support and decreased symptoms of illness.

Therefore, in order to start breaking the old patterns and habits of the subconscious, it's essential to harness the power of the conscious mind and the power of positive thinking. It won't be easy. It won't be quick. And you won't be perfect. You'll feel urges and temptations of old behavioral patterns during your journey. But the best thing to do is to *feel* those emotions fully. Be present. Let them pass without acting out externally. Don't confuse this method with suppressing them, though. Suppressing emotions means trying to ignore or numb the emotions. Instead, tune into your body and feel the emotion fully. Train your conscious mind to refrain from action. This is the epitome of free will and the most important decision you can make in the present moment because we all know how messy it gets when our beach ball splashes everyone around us.

Healthy Habits: Love

Cultivating self-love takes time and patience. It starts with accepting the present moment as it is and loving it unconditionally, regardless of the underlying emotion it elicits. Accept and embrace. Once we start to live in the present and appreciate each passing moment, we can begin the hard work of breaking the subconscious programming and behavioral patterns that make us feel like we're living our lives in a hamster wheel. The following healthy habits illustrate the true power of free will and potential for change, and will help you change destructive behavioral patterns. You can evolve. You can choose love.

1. Present Moment Breathing

Living in the present is harder than it sounds. In fact, for most of us it's nearly impossible. Completely in the moment? What is that? Our minds have been dominated by past regrets and future fears for as long as we can remember. A great way to reconnect with the present moment, though, is through the breath. The breath is the only thing that is completely in the present moment—always. By bringing awareness to the breath during the act of breathing, you can re-teach your mind and body to live in the present.

For this breathing practice, make sure to inhale large and audible breaths. At full inhalation, let go of the breath without any pauses. Once fully exhaled, begin inhaling again immediately without pause. The goal is to create one single long breath without pause for the entire five-, 10- or even 15-minute breathing meditation. Every time you practice this habit of reconnecting with your breath, involve the mental and physical aspects of your awareness so both your mind and body experience the present moment. Make your breath audible so that you both hear it and feel it. This will occupy your physical body and mind during the process.

Intentional, conscious and deep breathing may seem like an easy task, but it takes significant effort and concentration. It's uncomfortable at times because the mind will race. Fight the urge to stop and resist the impulse to fidget. Set your alarm for the allotted time and sit completely still in a comfortable position. Whatever emotion, thought or feeling that may arise during the breathing practice is fine, just be with it until it passes. Don't stop your breathing practice until the alarm goes off. Most of the discomfort is due to your mind's inability to be completely present. This could be new and uncharted territory, but by intentionally practicing living in the moment with your breathing practice, it will be easier to access in everyday life.

If nothing else, you will enjoy a few moments of mental stillness when the voice in your head is completely switched off. It will feel euphoric! Be open-minded and try it for yourself. If you enjoy the results, it may serve you well to pick up Michael Brown's *The Presence Process*. Much of the insight provided throughout this chapter regarding the importance of experiencing the present moment as it is was inspired by his writing and works.

2. Create Your Sankalpa

A Sankalpa is similar to a positive affirmation, but it is much deeper and more significant in its meaning. It's a personal resolution that helps define and create the life you're meant to enjoy and embrace. Let's break it down. *Kalpa* means 'vow' or 'promise'. *San* refers to an association with the highest truth. *Sankalpa*, then, is a commitment that you make as a cornerstone to support your highest truth.

Make your resolution at the beginning of the day when you're calm and your day is about to begin. Calm, because this is the state of mind you must be in for the words to truly penetrate your subconscious. If you're stressed, your encouraging, guiding and uplifting words and intentions will do nothing.

Carry your Sankalpa with you throughout the day and repeat it as often as you like, both in your heads and out loud when appropriate. The Sankalpa is not about material or superficial affirmations. Choose statements and affirmations that will transform your life physically, mentally, emotionally and spiritually. Some examples of Sankalpas are *I am a positive force for the evolution of others, I recognize my personal power and potential,* or *I am a student of life; I teach with my actions.*

Remember that change doesn't happen overnight, especially the lifelong change that you're after. Conscious reprogramming takes a long time and requires consistent and intentional practice. Choose a Sankalpa that represents the very core of your being, and don't judge the success of your positive affirmation if you don't see immediate benefits in your life. Keep it as your personal mantra and recite it to yourself when you need to hear those reaffirming words.

3. Date Night

When you date someone you romantically like, you spend time and effort trying to impress the other person by being on your best behavior, focusing on their needs and making sure they're happy throughout the process. Well, it's time to show that same tender love and care to yourself. When was the last time you took yourself on a date and pampered yourself?

It's important to treat yourself with the same respect you treat others. Some people jump from failed relationship to failed relationship without ever realizing that the real problem is that they don't really love themselves. They look for external sources of validation and approval in the form of a relationship with someone else. What they need to do first is turn their search for love towards themselves. If you find time to appreciate yourself, you may find that you will attract higher quality relationships with others too. These seemingly small acts of self-compassion and kindness towards oneself promote self-regulation of health related behaviors, making you healthier and better able to cope with life's many stressful situations.[13]

We spend so much time and energy focusing on pleasing others that we simply forget to recharge the source of that energy: our souls. It's only when you nourish your own mind, body and soul that you will have the internal resources necessary to continue giving to others and creating positive change to those around you. This is a simple yet fun concept that will dramatically improve your health and mental wellbeing. Remove disturbances like your cell phone, schedule a time when you can pick yourself up, and take yourself on a date. Solo.

4. Keep a Gratitude Journal

One of the unhealthiest habitual recipes for depression is comparing your own situation to someone else's. In a world where social media websites allow us to peer into the lives of our friends from a distance, we're provided with endless opportunities to compare our lives to theirs. But the problem is that you're comparing their highlight reel to your behind-the-scenes. Very few people advertise their struggles, hardships and pitfalls. Can you imagine if people shared their every emotionally charged moment on social media channels? Most just publish their accomplishments (or baby photos). You don't see what went into the events being posted on their Facebook walls. Stop comparing yourself with them, then, because it creates an endless cycle of comparison that leaves you bitter with your own situation.

Keep your mind focused on the positive aspects of your own life. There's so much to be thankful for, even if it's as simple as knowing you have all of your meals for the day. Keeping an attitude of appreciation will improve your health. Dr. Robert Emmons, a leading researcher in the growing field of 'positive psychology', found through his research that people who are grateful are more likely to engage in complementary health behaviors like exercising more and eating healthier, which in turns improves cognitive function, makes them feel happier, and even creates stronger immune systems.[14] Measureable physiological benefits like higher levels of HDL, heart rate variability and lower levels of blood pressure are also associated with people who practice gratitude.[15]

When you wake up or before you go to sleep, paint your mental landscape with positive thinking using a gratitude journal. Everyone, regardless of circumstance and situation, can find something in their lives to be thankful for. The more you search, the more you'll find too. Keep a journal. Write down the things you're grateful for. Cultivate an attitude of gratitude by showing appreciation, and consciously be thankful for the positive areas of your life.

5. Connect Physically

Humans are social creatures and need physical connection to thrive. In fact, it's essential in every stage of life, particularly in the early years when a child is developing cognitive awareness and emotional capacity. One hallmark study out of Romania found that despite having all of their basic needs met, orphans who lacked physical touch had increased rates of developmental problems, immune system dysfunction and behavioral problems.[16] But touch is also important as we get older and engage with relationships with other people, regardless of whether those relationships are grounded on sexual intimacy. We need human touch to be healthy.

Next time you're feeling down, don't reach for the medicine cabinet; reach for another person. It's time to invade someone's personal space. Preferably, it's someone you're already intimate with. Researchers have found that popping your personal space bubble and hugging others impacts hormone production—namely oxytocin, the happy hormone—and lowers blood pressure.[17] Hugging is an investment that keeps on giving! And the more frequent the hugs, the greater the health benefits.[18] If you're single, hug a stranger. (It's probably best you ask permission first, though.)

Truly Sustainable Living

"Man will survive as he reprograms readily to that which the ecosystem needs of him so long as he does not forget who is serving who. What is done well for the ecosystem is good for man. However, the cultures that say only what is good for man is good for nature may pass and be forgotten like the rest."
– Howard Odum

"All larger organisms, including ourselves, are living testimonies to the fact that destructive practices do not work in the long run. In the end, the aggressors always destroy themselves, making way for others who know how to cooperate and get along. Life is much less a competitive struggle for survival than a triumph of cooperation and creativity." – Fritjof Capra

If you knew David 12 months ago, you'd be forgiven for double-taking if you passed him in the street today. David is absolutely unrecognizable. He has simply transformed his life by swapping destructive and addictive lifestyles and habits with proactive and life-sustaining habits based on the six Healthy Lifestyle Principles: Real Food, Movement, Rest and Relaxation, Lifelong Learning, Community and Love. David now eats a healthy diet primarily made up of real food, and he can confidently and quickly identify which food adds to or detracts from his health. Exercise has become an essential part of his daily life too, because he now understands that regular movement and circulation are vital for optimal health. He's implemented a good sleep routine to give his body enough time to rest and recuperate, then wake up ready to tackle life all over again the following day. He no longer watches TV, instead preferring to spend his free time outdoors, reading a good book, hanging out with friends and family, or learning new hobbies. David barely recognizes himself any more—but that's a good thing.

The changes in his life aren't just limited to increased energy and improved quality of life either. David's also discovered an intellectual curiosity that he didn't know existed. During his Lifestyle Transformation program, David realized that health is a lifelong journey, not a final destination; a dynamic process that ebbs and flows with each lifestyle decision; a process that constantly evolves and improves; but a process that's also very vulnerable if disregarded for long periods of time. David has experienced nothing but excitement and revelation as he's learned more about health and wellness, researched his questions and experimented on himself. He has 100% owned his lifestyle transformation from day one, producing a new and improved version of himself that's barely recognizable in the mirror, and even less recognizable in his thoughts and behaviors.

David's Lifestyle Transformation has had unforeseen consequences too. What started as a selfish desire to improve his personal health quickly changed into something much bigger. Gradually David discovered the intimate connection between his health, the environment and even future generations. His healthy lifestyle wasn't just about himself anymore. His daily decisions impacted not only the health of people around him, but also the natural environment at large. He began to connect the dots.

David realized that choosing organic was more than just a healthy food choice for himself; by doing so he effectively cast a vote to support sustainable agriculture practices that focus on the long-term health and fertility of the soil, the most important natural resource we need to grow food. Organic farmers don't use synthetic chemical inputs like fertilizers, pesticides and herbicides, but instead implement farming strategies that work *with* nature's inherent biodiversity rather than against it. Choosing to buy his fresh produce from organic farmers ensured that David supported the future of his natural environment too.

Though he didn't have children of his own yet, David began to understand that when it was time, his children's health *tomorrow* would be impacted by his diet *today*. When he bought from local food producers, he helped keep wealth within his own community, thus contributing to the community's long-term resiliency and viability. In his mind, every time he made a food decision or even ate a meal, he cast a vote with the almighty dollar. Which agricultural systems did David want to provide food for his children? Organic methods that produce healthier food and preserve the environment in the process; or industrial practices that prioritize maximum economic profits over environmental awareness, subsequently resulting in socioeconomic and ecological destruction? David never labeled himself as an environmentalist, but the choice was simple. If he had to spend his hard-earned cash on food, he would support not only his own health but the health of the world around him.

David learned an important lesson when he began connecting the dots. You don't just eat for yourself. Your food choices impact the environment, your local community, your health, even the genes of future generations. Because when you eat, you eat for all humankind.

Eating for All Humankind

The 'butterfly effect' is a concept that attempts to link seemingly small changes in one place or time with drastic alterations in a later place or time. Edward Lorenz, the pioneer of the chaos theory, coined and named the effect after providing an example of a hurricane being formed as a direct result of a distant butterfly flapping its wings several weeks prior to the hurricane's formation. While at first sight these two events seem completely unrelated and isolated from one another, Lorenz said they could be intimately connected. The inference that can be drawn from this concept is that nothing exists in isolation. Everything is connected.

Even Hollywood filmmakers jumped on board with this concept. In the movie *The Butterfly Effect*, Evan discovers that he has the power to go back in time to revisit moments in his childhood and actually change what happened. Despite his best intentions to save his childhood sweetheart from being molested by her father and harassed by her brother, his small intrusions on the past have drastic impacts on everyone's future. Every action he takes leads to unforeseen consequences, to the point that Evan becomes disheartened and desperate for resolution. In one reality, Evan ends up disabled. In another, his childhood sweetheart gets into a relationship with Evan's best friend. The Director's Cut of the movie ends with Evan concluding that the main cause of his loved one's problems in every one of the parallel timelines he experiences is actually himself. Evan thus travels back in time to when he was still in his mother's womb, and strangles himself with the umbilical cord. Evan dies knowing that he saved his childhood sweetheart, despite not allowing himself to actually do life with her.

Although not quite as dramatic, your daily lifestyle decisions also create a quasi-butterfly effect. The seemingly small decisions like *what should I eat for lunch?* or *where should I buy groceries?* actually impact the environment as well as the very fabric of our socioeconomic infrastructure. When you sit down at the table and your meal consists of genetically modified food that has been grown by large agribusinesses or food conglomerates and treated with pesticides, you directly support the destructive environmental and socioeconomic practices of these businesses—whether you mean to or not.

The use of GMO technology in agriculture is a great example of how something that has great potential to be beneficial to the world as a whole, is instead used as a tool for power and economic gain for a small group of people at the expense of everyone else. Some GMO technologies claim to have the potential to protect against insect damage, reduce the land needed for agriculture, conserve natural resources like water, or allow plants to grow in harsh ecological environments and soils that otherwise could not support plant life at all. We have to assume that long-term testing has confirmed the safety of the crops, both for human consumption and for the broader ecosystem, however when we tinker with the laws of nature it's imperative to be cautious and objective. As human populations continue to rise, some GMO technologies might actually add to our sustainable downfall, despite claiming to support longevity.

Unfortunately, many of the GMO technologies hinder some environmental, social and economic aspects of sustainability. In terms of environmental sustainability, GMO agricultural technologies seriously threaten agricultural and natural systems biodiversity, both of which provide the very foundation of sustainability.[1,2,3] There are two components to biodiversity. The first is genetic diversity, which is a measure of diversity within a species. The second is ecosystem diversity, which is the number of different species in a defined region or area. In both cases, you will find the heightened use of monocultures to be the core of the problem and perhaps the biggest threat to agricultural and natural systems biodiversity, with GMOs primarily impacting genetic biodiversity.

A monoculture is a field planted or filled with genetically similar plants or animals. Monocultures inherently contain very little genetic diversity due to the dominant genetic characteristics of specialized varieties (also known as 'cultivars'). GMO technology takes the problem of monocultures one step further, because all of the plants or animals within a given variety are genetically identical and tightly controlled by the seed producer. The corn industry is a perfect example of this, since nearly 90% of corn in the United States is genetically modified.

When genes are more diverse and able to adapt to specific ecological and cultural circumstances over generations, they become more resilient. Look to the dog world for proof: while mutts aren't always the ideal puppy choice, they do have fewer and less extreme health problems than purebred dogs that come from one lineage. Crops are no different. Crops with reduced genetic diversity (the purebreds of the agricultural world) are often more vulnerable to climatic extremes and attacks by pests and diseases than their non-GMO counterparts (the mutts), simply because they haven't been given the opportunity to adapt to the environment where they're grown. While GMOs may protect against a certain set of threats determined in the laboratory, they may be unable to cope with the drought, floods, heat, cold, pests and diseases encountered on any given farm. More importantly, the biological threats that they've been genetically developed and modified to protect against may evolve to be resistant to the genetic alterations, in much the same way that mosquitoes often begin to adapt to the chemicals in mosquito repellent, making the technology obsolete until a new short-term modification is developed.

Thanks to traits carefully predetermined in the lab and field trials of the company that owns the seed, crops are never given the opportunity to adapt to their on-farm environments. They're never given the chance to reproduce naturally and adapt to that specific farm and the variables that make it unique, like soil quality, species diversity and climate. In fact, farmers sign contracts that forbid them to reuse these seeds in subsequent plantings.

Finally, GMOs can also overwhelm heirloom and indigenous species. Unprecedented numbers of native species and heirloom varieties of plants are endangered in our era, so it is critical for us to protect both natural and agricultural biodiversity through our food choices. This issue extends not only to terrestrial food production but also to all types of aquatic environments.[4] Protecting our portfolio of diverse life is similar to keeping an investment portfolio open and diverse. Biodiversity protects against risk and keeps ecosystems strong and resilient against unexpected environmental and ecological changes.

It's not just the environment that GMO has negative effects on. GMO technology also impacts socioeconomic aspects of sustainability. Rather than a tool for improving food security, GMOs are used as tools for power and economic profits. A small handful of companies like Monsanto, DuPont and Syngenta own the patents associated with GMOs and severely restrict their use. Farmer sovereignty is rigorously threatened when farmers are forced into economically unfavorable and unreasonable practices imposed by large agribusinesses. Only the largest food producers are economically viable, primarily thanks to governmental subsidies rather than farming effectiveness and efficiency.

Additionally, these large agribusinesses possess the power— and practice it frequently—to sue farmers whose fields have been contaminated with GMO seed,[5] even if the contamination resulted from unintentional drift from neighboring farms. Due to the structure and high cost of the court system, farmers stand little chance in courts due to lack of funds and time to fight these long and drawn-out legal battles. Small farmers, after all, must tend to their land to survive. At the core of GMO technology is corporate power and attempts to maintain economic strangleholds on the industry. Even within the socioeconomic landscape, politically and economically powerful companies that own GMO patents adversely impact diversity by eliminating competition, effectively creating an oligarchy.

Aside from being GMO, the food on your plate was also probably sprayed with chemical pesticides, which bring their own set of environmental and social consequences. The people who grow food that's sprayed with pesticides are often exposed to highly toxic pesticides themselves, which have been linked to many health problems, most notably birth defects and reproductive issues.[6,7,8,9] Due to lax regulations, the usage of banned or severely restricted chemicals not to mention a lack of proper education around handling pesticides, exposure to pesticides and its associated health problems are significantly more prevalent in developing countries.[10] We are culturally and geographically separated from the health consequences associated with growing our food because we don't actually grow it ourselves, so in turn very few of us understand the social ramifications of pesticide use on local populations in developing countries. Consumption of pesticide residue has also been linked to neurodevelopment and growth issues[11], as well as elevated rates of chronic diseases such as different types of cancers, diabetes, neurodegenerative disorders, Alzheimer's and reproductive disorders.[12] Unbeknownst to the eater, their food choice may be carrying lots of bad pesticide karma.

As discussed previously, ecosystems thrive when there is biodiversity because a wide varieties of species and organisms keep the system in balance and more resilient against disease, pests, and extreme environmental changes. Simply put, an ecosystem's strength rests on its diversity. On the other hand, monocultures are inherently more susceptible to pests and disease—ironically enough. When large-scale farming operations rely on a single crop to produce and perform, that crop becomes more vulnerable and lacks the protection that would have otherwise existed if it had grown within a diverse environment. Instead of natural protection provided by other organisms, monocultures rely on external inputs such as pesticides and herbicides. Unfortunately, this protection comes at the expense of the ecological community surrounding the monoculture. Amphibian populations are declining worldwide at an alarming rate, with pesticides being among the proposed causes.[13] More importantly, bee populations worldwide are declining, with significant blame being cast upon pesticide exposure.[14] *But what's so important about bees?* you ask. Agriculturally speaking, a lot. Many varieties of nuts and vegetation such as alfalfa, apple, cantaloupe, pumpkin and sunflower require pollination from bees to continue to produce. In fact, one in every three mouthfuls of food you eat depends on honeybee pollination.[15] The continued decline in bees should strike significant alarm bells and put into question the agricultural practices currently dominating the industrialized food system.

It's easy to ignore or simply not realize the practices responsible for putting food on your plate, because you're not the person doing it. The food you eat has a story of its own that needs to be known and understand. It's both an empowering and frightening experience when you first realize the extent to which your individual lifestyle impacts the world. Like the Hollywood movie *The Butterfly Effect* illustrates, small decisions today can create huge impacts tomorrow. Unlike the movie, however, the lifestyle decisions you make today have more predictable outcomes in the future.

If you eat foods that have been genetically modified or grown with pesticides, you directly support the agricultural practices that destroy not just the human body, but also socioeconomic aspects of society. The simple practice of eating is more than just personal health and welfare. It's about environmental sustainability and social equality too. Even if you're still not convinced that organic food is better for you than the alternative, know that supporting the agricultural practices that grow organic food means you also support farming methods that are better for the environment. Organic practices focus on the long-term health of farming system,[16] refrain from using environmentally destructive fertilizers,[17] humanely handle their livestock and keep their products antibiotic-free, and preserve the biological activity of the soil.[18] Organic is more than a label or title. If you pay attention to the food on your plate, you can hear its story. What story is your food telling you?

That's not all; even choosing to buy organic food locally rather than from out of town is better for everyone in the long run. On a socioeconomic level, buying cheaper foods from non-local sources has of the most significant butterfly effects on local communities. This seems like common sense, yet many of us still prefer convenience and price over long-term community vision. On the flipside, more dollars that circulate from local transactions translate into stronger local businesses, more jobs, more wealth and thus a healthier local economy.[19] This is an economic phenomenon known as the multiplier effect, which means that one dollar spent locally reaps local rewards several times over. Some economists have even estimated the impact to be roughly seven times over.[20] That means every dollar you spend at a local business represents a $7 benefit for your local community. Buying from large businesses like Walmart rather than local small businesses may result in a smaller cost to your wallet at first, but in the long run it can result in less wealth for the community as whole. Some studies of small communities have shown that where Walmart appears, poverty rates actually rise over time.[21] Whether this relationship is direct or causal remains to be unknown, but the implication is that dollars that would have circulated locally, thus benefitting multiple local businesses and people, are instead removed from the community and invested into distant shareholders and foreign manufacturers and producers.

Buying locally doesn't just support economic sustainability either. When local money is spent elsewhere, economically poor communities also become unhealthier and lack access, resources, assistance and education to improve their situations. Poverty and ill-health are intimately connected. As poverty increases, so too do medical costs, impoverishment and inequality.[22] Obesity rates are highest among populations with the highest poverty rates.[23] The primary factors contributing to this social phenomenon are the relative affordability of energy-dense and unhealthy foods[24] and the subsequent reduction of access to healthy and nutritious foods.[25] Buying locally is an investment in the long-term health and sustainability of the local community and the people living within it.

...

We're constantly told that, by nature, mankind manipulates ways to get the greatest pleasure for the least amount of effort. This is often the simpler, cheaper and more convenient way to live life. But what if we were to choose another way? What if we started to second-guess those instinctive responses and rise above them? A new way of thinking about the world would mean small sacrifices today so that everyone benefits tomorrow—small sacrifices that are hardly felt at the individual level, but are obviously seen at the collective level.

As you read this you may be thinking *how can a single person impact the food system alone?* The truth is, the food system we know today was actually formed by that very same mentality. Our modern food system is the butterfly effect of collectively choosing convenience over quality. It was self-created by many people who independently made small choices, but failed to realize their choices would combine to create drastic change over time. The very same process will be responsible for reshaping and redirecting the food system that our children will inherit. Change happens one meal at a time. More specifically, it happens one dollar at a time.

Your dietary decisions contribute to the world that you will live in for years to come. Until our socioeconomic systems change, the future is shaped by where you spend your dollars *today*. With every buying decision you make, you cast a vote that is arguably as powerful as our over-arching political system. Currently, many of the farm legislative and policy structures strongly favor the large agribusinesses that are directly responsible for the destructive agricultural practices we see today. Politics takes a long time to change. Too long. Buying decisions, on the other hand, are instant. That's why voting with your dollars is every bit as important as voting at the polls.

Maybe it's hard to comprehend the power of the individual, but each and every one of us plays an important role in creating the world we will leave behind for future generations. One of the simplest yet most profound ways to impact this world is with the food choices you make. Once we realize the wider effects our food choices have on our futures, it becomes our inherent responsibility to remember that we're not only eating for ourselves, we're eating for all humankind.

Genetic Sustainability: The 4th Pillar

Sustainability can mean different things to different people. What most sustainability advocates can agree upon, though, is that sustainability is made up of the integration of social, environmental and economic factors. These are commonly called the three pillars of sustainability, and are often used to assess and compare proposed projects and initiatives for change. All three pillars must be taken into account and analyzed, and rightfully so. Until our economic system completely changes, sustainability *should* reconcile people, plants and profits. Because the focus of this book has been on an individual's personal health, a fourth pillar of sustainability becomes relevant and deserves a continued discussion: human genetics.

We can all agree that our lifestyle plays the most important role when determining our health, both now and as we age. If you focus your life on health, you'll be rewarded with energy, vitality and longevity. If you choose to neglect your health, you'll met be with the opposite: an increased need for medical interventions, chronic disease and a shorter lifespan. But your personal health, as important as it is, is not the only thing on the line here. What needs to be considered with every lifestyle choice is that those decisions impact you on the most fundamental of levels: your genetics. Let's revisit the poker analogy from the introduction of this book.

In poker, you start with a five-card hand dealt to you by the dealer. After viewing your hand and strategizing how to best improve it, you're given the opportunity to discard cards you don't want and replace them with cards you draw at random from the top of the deck. The game is based largely on probability and statistics, with a little bit luck thrown in for good measure. The best five-card hand wins the game.

Your genes are similar in nature. When you were born you were dealt a genetic hand that you had no control over. Nonetheless, your genes are your starting poker hand, and you can either choose to give up or play the game. Unlike the game of poker in which you draw from the remaining deck of cards, though, your genes are not left up to chance or probability. Instead, you have a choice. You can consciously improve your hand, or you can make it worse. The game of genetic poker lasts your entire lifetime, and you change your genetic destiny with the lifestyle choices you make.

Food, as it turns out, is more than just nutrients broken down for use as fuel, structure and energy. The food you eat is similar to drawing cards from the deck during a game of poker. Yes, food changes your poker hand. We literally share genetic information with some of the food we eat. Genetically speaking, the food you eat directly influences your genetic expression[26] and can even damage your genes.[27] This takes healthy eating to a much greater level of importance. Here's how the process works. MicroRNA are tiny molecules in the food we eat. They're responsible for regulation of gene expression, are involved in most biological processes, and are picked up by the digestive system and transferred into our own cells when we eat food.[28] Subsequently, they bind to chromosomes within our cells and alter the expression of genes. *You are what you eat* takes on a whole new meaning when you consider this phenomenon.

What this means for the food you choose to eat is paramount. Human bodies have evolved over millions of years to eat real food—whole, natural and unprocessed. However, emerging food production and processing technologies have made genetic changes to food that would have otherwise taken thousands of years—if at all. Their food products are designed more for their economic implications rather than the long-term implications when consumed by humans. There are no long-term studies of how microRNA from genetically modified foods impact the human genome and genetic expression. We do, however, know that nature's originals have been working just fine for millions of years.

It's not just food that influences human genetics, either. Not surprisingly, if you regularly exercise, your genes will benefit.[29] Even short-term exercise programs have been shown to protect your genes.[30] On the other hand, if you're chronically stressed, your genes will be negatively damaged.[31] A short restorative meditation session can be a long-term investment in your genetic health. When it comes to nature vs. nurture, we're not at the mercy of our genes. In fact, they are at the mercy of our lifestyle—and so too are our children. The game of genetic poker never stops.

If our lifestyle plays an important role in the genetic health within our lifetime, then it makes sense that they play a role in the genes we pass on to the next generation. Since most parents want what's best for their children and wish them a life better than their own, it is the parents who are in the ultimate position of power when it comes to making that wish a reality. We contribute to the overall genetic health of our offspring, and it depends significantly on how we choose to live our lives. If a parent's diet lacks the adequate nutrients the body needs to thrive, their children's genes will suffer too.[32,33] This goes for both parents too, not just mom.[34] Diet even contributes to the genetic susceptibility and inherent risk of chronic disease in offspring.[35] Leading a life focused on health will benefit the genes of your children. A life of neglecting health will have the opposite effect. Just how broad and far-reaching are these genetic implications? The answer may surprise you. Recent research shows that our lifestyles impact our genes for several generations, not just for our children. Persistent and chronic stress in your lifetime will impact not only children,[36] but also your grandchildren.[37,38]

The importance of keeping your genes healthy is obvious. People with healthier genes lead healthier lives. They're more resilient to disease, less likely to encounter chronic disease during their lifetime, and more likely to lead lives filled with energy and vitality. The individual, however, is not the only benefactor of healthy genes; the wider society is too. With healthcare costs amounting to roughly $2.5 billion annually (nearly 18% of the total US economy),[39] it is in society's best interest to take the notion of genetic sustainability seriously.

As our genes become weaker, so too does our resilience to disease and ability to adapt to sudden environmental changes. In other words, as our genetic health as a species deteriorates, so too do our chances for long-term sustainability. Taking responsibility and action towards our personal health and wellbeing may be the most important socioeconomic decision you can make.

What's best for our personal health is best for the environment, our socioeconomic infrastructures, our genes and, of course, future generations. It's all connected. Selfishly choosing to focus on your own health may be the most selfless act of all in the end. The more you invest in your personal health now, the more you will end up giving back to the world around you in the future. You can begin to change the world simply by building the foundation of your life around the six Healthy Lifestyle Principles: Real Food, Movement, Rest and Relaxation, Life Learning, Community and Love. All it takes is focusing on and changing one habit at a time, and this book has provided you with enough for an entire year. That is precisely what the final chapter of this book provides: a 52-week program utilizing the healthy habits from each chapter. With your knowledge of the six Healthy Lifestyle Principles, it's time for your Lifestyle Transformation.

Lifestyle Transformation

"Every day do something that will inch you closer to a better tomorrow."
– Doug Firebaugh

"The best thing about the future is that it comes only one day at a time."
– Abraham Lincoln

When you ask people why they don't already lead a healthy lifestyle, they often reply that it's too hard or it requires too much time. In reality, it actually has nothing to do with either of those excuses.

Healthy living is easy and doesn't require any effort at all if it's already your current lifestyle. It's the change that comes with choosing a healthy lifestyle over an unhealthy one that can be too hard and take up too much time, not the healthy lifestyle itself. Even though it might seem pedantic, it's that slight difference in thinking that's absolutely critical for you to understand.

People become so accustomed to the status quo of their lives that change seems difficult, uncomfortable and impossible. Thinking about how much change would have to be made in order to lead a healthy lifestyle can be overwhelming, to say the least. Their current habits are so engrained, they can't imagine being able to break all of them let alone just one. But if you want to create your very own Lifestyle Transformation, just like David did, you need to start understanding how your underlying habits work and, more importantly, how they were formed in the first place. Because that's how you're going to break them.

How many times have you set out to get healthier? Probably more than you can count on your two hands. It's the same pattern every time:

1. Feel motivated.
2. Set goal.
3. Get started.
4. Cheat.
5. Lose momentum.
6. Forget about goal. Feel like a failure.
7. Wash. Rinse. Repeat and start back at step number one some other time in the future.

It sounds familiar, doesn't it. I also bet that every time you repeat this series of steps, it gets harder and harder to get to step number one. Why?

It's simple actually. Every time you fail to follow through with your healthy lifestyle change, you start to associate the pain and discouragement from your failed attempt with healthy living. Every time you begin to think about changing your lifestyle, you remember how you felt last time and assume you'll feel the same this time around. After all, why is this time going to be any different?

So you stay where you are. It's comfortable, easier, less painful. When you finally sum up the courage to face your fears of pain and failure, you try again. But you experience the same results. And this time, the association of pain and failure with healthy living grows even stronger, until you finally throw up the white flag and decide trying is just not worth it any more. *It's not my fault. It's my genes. It runs in my family. I can't do anything about it.*

It's normal to protect yourself from pain and discouragement; your brain created biological protective mechanisms so you can actually function normally. But this is also why change is so hard. Unhealthy habits have simply become so engrained in your life that breaking them literally seems impossible to do. Bad habits become your default programming.

But all of that ends now.

You may have failed in the past, but today is different. With the right knowledge, tools, motivation and system of accountability, healthy change is just around the corner. You've just got to grab it.

The first step to lifelong change is becoming aware of the problem. You've already done that. Habits are your problem. Bad habits have become so deeply programmed in your behavioral patterns, you don't even realize they exist. That's why when you set out to eat healthy in the past, you blinked and found a donut in your mouth without even thinking about it. Someone else *must* have put that there.

But that person is not you anymore. You know the problem boils down to your bad habits. You don't have to be hard on yourself anymore because you know what you're dealing with is normal and, more importantly, changeable. You can get rid of bad habits and substitute them with good habits with the same logic and approach. You can make healthy living your default behavior. In the face of adversity, the healthy choice will eventually feel like the natural choice.

The only requirement is your unwavering desire for positive and healthy change. If you are determined to change, that you have no choice except to change, then the habits of the Lifestyle Transformation Program will provide you with the direct path to precisely that. David did it. Now it's your turn. Welcome to YOUR Lifestyle Transformation.

...

The Lifestyle Transformation Program is the best and most effective way to implement healthy habits outlined throughout *Million Ways to Live*. This program provides a structure that is measureable, manageable and sustainable, by implementing **one habit every two weeks** over the course of a year.

Changing your entire lifestyle takes time, focus and patience. Your bad habits will be slowly and effectively replaced by healthy and proactive habits that build upon your foundation of health. Some of the healthy habits won't stick after the two weeks, while others will become as second nature as brushing your teeth. But as you progress through the program, you will start to build a healthy lifestyle from the ground up, one habit at a time. Want a sneak preview at the future you? Here are a few things you'll enjoy as a result of your commitment to health:

- Improved energy
- Improved body composition
- Better digestion
- Improved resistance to illnesses

- Increased sex drive
- Better sex
- Improved skin quality
- Improved work productivity
- Improved mental health

Although every person is unique, the progression of habits and the order in which they are implemented is consistent with bad habits most people in everyday society share. Not surprisingly, the first habits focus on Real Food and Movement. In the modern day world of convenience and sedentary lifestyles, this is the area we all need the most help with. If you want to follow your own path, feel free to implement the habits in the order of your choosing. But know that this program was structured and organized in this order for a reason.

Accountability

In order to help with accountability, the Lifestyle Transformation Program begins with filling out a personal health contract. Take a picture of it on your cell phone and make it the background. Pin it up on your wall at work. Tape it to your bathroom mirror. **Read it aloud every morning and night.**

Your health is the most important investment you can make. Remind yourself everyday so you can keep your motivation levels up. Don't let your favorite tried-and-true excuses win the mental battle for the behaviors you choose to make. **Take responsibility for your health and your success**—because no one else is going to.

Another way to increase accountability is to get other people involved. Go public with your goals by telling people about what you're trying to do. You may lose some friends along the way, but you'll also make new like-minded friends who will help you with your goals. As a group, you can then keep each other accountable and focused on your goals. Remember, in community there is strength, which is exactly why Community is one of the Healthy Lifestyle Principles. And if you need help finding a supportive community, you can do the Lifestyle Transformation program with the LEAF community (www.leaflifestyle.com), which provides you with professional coaching and guidance as you build your healthy lifestyle.

Tracking Progress

Each habit has its own sheet which gives you the details, tips and tricks to get you started. While these suggestions are great starting points, I encourage you to explore different options and try anything that's in line with both the Healthy Lifestyle Principle and the specific habit that's being taught for the two weeks.

Each habit sheet also has areas to check compliance. The more you comply, the faster and more significant the results you'll enjoy. 100% compliance will produce much greater results than 70% compliance, for example. The goal is to comply 80% to 90% of the time throughout the duration of the one-year program. And remember, success begets success. When you stay committed, focus and strict, your healthy lifestyle becomes easy and effortless. If you find yourself complying 60% or less, it's probably time to step in front of a mirror and give yourself a bit of a pep talk.

In order to track progress in a quantitative and objective manner, weight, BMI, circumference measurements and body fat percentage will be measured and tracked throughout the Lifestyle Transformation Program. Before you start each habit, weigh yourself and calculate your BMI, circumference measurements and body fat percentage (visit www.leaflifestyle.com for help). At the end of each two-week period, weigh yourself again and re-calculate all three metrics. These figures will serve as the starting figures for the next habit.

They say a picture is worth a thousand words, so grab a camera or use a cell phone to take some before photos. You may not like what you see, but a visual representation of what you used to look like will make you so much more proud of yourself once you reach your goals. You need three photos: facing the camera, from the side, and from the back. Make sure you get your whole body in the shot. No one has to see the pictures except you. When you finish this journey, your after photos will capture a snapshot of what your success looks like. What you *feel* will be much more significant, but pictures nonetheless provide great comparisons and memories.

It's time to start your Lifestyle Transformation. Step one: fill out the personal health contract that will finalize and formalize your commitment to your health.

Lifestyle Transformation - Personal Health Contract

I, _____, hereby reclaim responsibility of my own health. In order to do this, I will complete the Million Ways to Live Lifestyle Transformation Program by committing to the following:

- I will not let small mistakes or slip-ups allow me to stop my progress. I will not create negative self-talk and convince myself that I am stupid, worthless or a lost cause. This kind of self-abuse is not healthy. No one is perfect. It's about progress, not perfection. In times of mental weakness, I will read this contract, create positive affirmations or reach out to my supporters for help and encouragement. **I will not allow myself to self-sabotage achieving the health I deserve as birthright.**

- I will not sacrifice my health progression in order to make other people happy. I know that when I am healthy, I will have more energy and vitality that can be used to help the world around me. When I am faced with a decision between my program and what my peers expect of me, **I will choose my health first and foremost.** I will compromise with friends, family and peers to create reasonable solutions that allow me to continue doing what I need to do for my own health and progress.

- I am personally responsible for both where my life is right now, and where my life is heading. **I take personal responsibility for all actions and behaviors from this point forward.** The degree of my success is up to no one but myself. If I break from the program, it is my conscious decision and I will be accountable for it, no one else.

I am committed to leading a healthier lifestyle because every aspect of my life will be better as a result. **I am motivated. I am committed. I am ready.**

To my health,

_____   _____

(signature)   (date)

Million Ways to Live

WEEK #: 1

HEALTHY LIFESTYLE PRINCIPLE: Real Food

HEALTHY HABIT: Conscious Consumption

LIFESTYLE TRANSFORMATION PROGRAM

HABIT DETAILS

Bring consciousness to an unconscious act. This will help you reconnect with your body and help prevent overeating by allowing your body's natural satiety hormones to do their job. Learn to listen to your body.

TIPS/TRICKS/SUGGESTIONS

- Chew each bite of food 30 times before swallowing
- Take two diaphragmatic breaths between bites
- Slow down
- Try to assess your satiety levels after each bite
- Stop at 80% full

HABIT COMPLIANCE: [   ] /14

Day 1	Day 2	Day 3	Day 4	Day 5	Day 6	Day 7
Y / N	Y / N	Y / N	Y / N	Y / N	Y / N	Y / N

Day 8	Day 9	Day 10	Day 11	Day 12	Day 13	Day 14
Y / N	Y / N	Y / N	Y / N	Y / N	Y / N	Y / N

NOTES/QUESTIONS/FEEDBACK:

BODY COMPOSITION PROGRESS:

Starting Weight:

Ending Weight:

Starting BF%:

Ending BF%:

Starting BMI:

Ending BMI:

CIRCUMFERENCE MEASUREMENTS:

	Starting	Ending
Neck		
Bicep		
Chest		
Waist		
Hips		
Thigh		

Healthy Habits Progress & Tracking Sheets

HEALTHY LIFESTYLE PRINCIPLE: Movement

HEALTHY HABIT: Daily Movement

LIFESTYLE TRANSFORMATION PROGRAM

HABIT DETAILS

Daily movement is the key to promoting circulation and keeping the body healthy. Make it a priority to move everyday. Small lifestyle decisions add up to a lot of movement throughout the day.

TIPS/TRICKS/SUGGESTIONS

- Park far away on trips to stores
- Take the stairs instead of the elevator
- Do a power walk during lunch at work
- Ride a bike to work
- Take a fitness class at the gym
- Do 30 minutes of strength training
- Go on a hike
- Do 20 minutes of yoga when you wake up

HABIT COMPLIANCE: [   ] /14

Day 1	Day 2	Day 3	Day 4	Day 5	Day 6	Day 7
Y / N	Y / N	Y / N	Y / N	Y / N	Y / N	Y / N

Day 8	Day 9	Day 10	Day 11	Day 12	Day 13	Day 14
Y / N	Y / N	Y / N	Y / N	Y / N	Y / N	Y / N

NOTES/QUESTIONS/FEEDBACK:

BODY COMPOSITION PROGRESS:

Starting Weight:	Ending Weight:

Starting BF%:	Ending BF%:

Starting BMI:	Ending BMI:

CIRCUMFERENCE MEASUREMENTS:

	Starting	Ending
Neck		
Bicep		
Chest		
Waist		
Hips		
Thigh		

Million Ways to Live

WEEK #: 5

HEALTHY LIFESTYLE PRINCIPLE: Love

HEALTHY HABIT: Present Moment Breathing

HABIT DETAILS

Connect with the present moment by connecting with your breath. Anything and everything that you feel is completely normal and valid. Be with it.

TIPS/TRICKS/SUGGESTIONS

1) Set your alarm so you don't worry about the time
2) Fight all urges to fidget
3) Audibly inhale and exhale (through the nose)
4) Just breathe

HABIT COMPLIANCE: [   ] /14

Day 1	Day 2	Day 3	Day 4	Day 5	Day 6	Day 7
Y / N	Y / N	Y / N	Y / N	Y / N	Y / N	Y / N

Day 8	Day 9	Day 10	Day 11	Day 12	Day 13	Day 14
Y / N	Y / N	Y / N	Y / N	Y / N	Y / N	Y / N

NOTES/QUESTIONS/FEEDBACK:

BODY COMPOSITION PROGRESS:

Starting Weight: **Ending Weight:**

Starting BF%:   **Ending BF%:**

Starting BMI: **Ending BMI:**

CIRCUMFERENCE MEASUREMENTS:

	Starting	Ending
Neck		
Bicep		
Chest		
Waist		
Hips		
Thigh		

Healthy Habits Progress & Tracking Sheets

WEEK #: 7

HEALTHY LIFESTYLE PRINCIPLE: Real Food

HEALTHY HABIT: Eat Real Food

**LIFESTYLE
TRANSFORMATION
PROGRAM**

HABIT DETAILS

Ditch the candy, chocolate, juice and junk food; opt instead for green veggies, smart carbs, lean proteins and healthy fats. The process starts with a kitchen makeover described in the Real Food chapter.

GENERAL MEAL SUGGESTIONS

Green Veggies (1/2 plate)	Smart Carbs (1/4 plate)	Lean Protein (1/4 plate)	Healthy Fat (optional)
• Spinach	• Quinoa	• Chicken or Beef	• Nuts (palmfu
• Kale	• Brown Rice	• Fish	• 1/4 Avocado
• Broccoli	• Sweet Potato	• Dairy	• Olive Oil
• Asparagus	• Fruit	• Legumes	• Coconut Oil

HABIT COMPLIANCE: [   ] /14

Day 1	Day 2	Day 3	Day 4	Day 5	Day 6	Day 7
Y / N	Y / N	Y / N	Y / N	Y / N	Y / N	Y / N

Day 8	Day 9	Day 10	Day 11	Day 12	Day 13	Day 14
Y / N	Y / N	Y / N	Y / N	Y / N	Y / N	Y / N

NOTES/QUESTIONS/FEEDBACK:

BODY COMPOSITION PROGRESS:

Starting Weight:

Ending Weight:

Starting BF%:

Ending BF%:

Starting BMI:

Ending BMI:

CIRCUMFERENCE MEASUREMENTS:

	Starting	Ending
Neck		
Bicep		
Chest		
Waist		
Hips		
Thigh		

207

Million Ways to Live

WEEK #: 9

HEALTHY LIFESTYLE PRINCIPLE: Rest & Relaxation

HEALTHY HABIT: Create a Sleep Routine

LIFESTYLE TRANSFORMATION PROGRAM

HABIT DETAILS

In today's modern world, we often don't get the sleep our bodies need to recover from the day and prepare for the next one. Create a four-step routine that you do every night before you go to bed, so your body begins to recognize when it's

TWO SAMPLE ROUTINES

1) Turn off all electronics 60 minutes before bedtime
2) Read for 20 minutes
3) Meditate for 10 minutes
4) Turn on a white noise app before going to sleep

1) Turn off the TV 30 minutes before bedtime
2) Write a journal entry reflecting on the day
3) Write down five things you are grateful for
4) Listen to a breathing meditation app for 10 minutes

HABIT COMPLIANCE: [   ] /14

Day 1	Day 2	Day 3	Day 4	Day 5	Day 6	Day 7
Y / N	Y / N	Y / N	Y / N	Y / N	Y / N	Y / N

Day 8	Day 9	Day 10	Day 11	Day 12	Day 13	Day 14
Y / N	Y / N	Y / N	Y / N	Y / N	Y / N	Y / N

NOTES/QUESTIONS/FEEDBACK:

BODY COMPOSITION PROGRESS:

Starting Weight:

Ending Weight:

Starting BF%:

Ending BF%:

Starting BMI:

Ending BMI:

CIRCUMFERENCE MEASUREMENTS:

	Starting	Ending
Neck		
Bicep		
Chest		
Waist		
Hips		
Thigh		

208

Healthy Habits Progress & Tracking Sheets

HEALTHY LIFESTYLE PRINCIPLE: Movement

HEALTHY HABIT: Exercise Intensification

LIFESTYLE TRANSFORMATION PROGRAM

HABIT DETAILS

You have to push yourself beyond your comfort zone to get results. Intensify your workout to reap the physiological benefits associated with higher intensity exercise. Intensify your workout 4 - 8 times. But don't forget daily movement!

TIPS/TRICKS/SUGGESTIONS

- Increase weight resistance
- Take a challenging fitness class
- Decrease rest time between sets
- Increase the number of sets
- Hire a fitness professional to help

HABIT COMPLIANCE: [   ] /8

Workout 1	Workout 2	Workout 3	Workout 4
Y / N	Y / N	Y / N	Y / N

Workout 5	Workout 6	Workout 7	Workout 8
Y / N	Y / N	Y / N	Y / N

NOTES/QUESTIONS/FEEDBACK:

BODY COMPOSITION PROGRESS:

Starting Weight:	Ending Weight:

Starting BF%:	Ending BF%:

Starting BMI:	Ending BMI:

CIRCUMFERENCE MEASUREMENTS:

	Starting	Ending
Neck		
Bicep		
Chest		
Waist		
Hips		
Thigh		

Million Ways to Live

WEEK #: 13

HEALTHY LIFESTYLE PRINCIPLE: Love

HEALTHY HABIT: Create Your Sankalpa

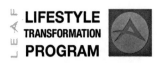

LIFESTYLE TRANSFORMATION PROGRAM

HABIT DETAILS

Create an intention or mantra that will guide and focus your mind in times of adversity, stress and frustration. Use only positive words. Keep it short. Repeat it to yourself every morning and night.

SAMPLES

1) I am at peace with myself.

2) I am empowered.

3) I enjoy perfect health.

4) I am already whole.

HABIT COMPLIANCE: [   ] /14

Day 1	Day 2	Day 3	Day 4	Day 5	Day 6	Day 7
Y / N	Y / N	Y / N	Y / N	Y / N	Y / N	Y / N

Day 8	Day 9	Day 10	Day 11	Day 12	Day 13	Day 14
Y / N	Y / N	Y / N	Y / N	Y / N	Y / N	Y / N

NOTES/QUESTIONS/FEEDBACK:

BODY COMPOSITION PROGRESS:

Starting Weight:

Ending Weight:

Starting BF%:

Ending BF%:

Starting BMI:

Ending BMI:

CIRCUMFERENCE MEASUREMENTS:

	Starting	Ending
Neck		
Bicep		
Chest		
Waist		
Hips		
Thigh		

Healthy Habits Progress & Tracking Sheets

WEEK #: 15

HEALTHY LIFESTYLE PRINCIPLE: Real Food

HEALTHY HABIT: Keep a Food Journal

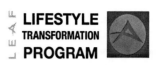

HABIT DETAILS

Write down everything you eat. Plan every meal ahead of time so you can schedule a diversity of foods into your diet and can time meals according with life demands (like workouts). Record how you feel after meals.

TIPS/TRICKS/SUGGESTIONS

- Use Instagram or your phone's camera to make logging easy. Write the food description in the caption
- Carry your journal with you and record everything you eat as you eat it
- Time meals around workouts and see which meals provide the best energy

HABIT COMPLIANCE: [   ] /14

Day 1	Day 2	Day 3	Day 4	Day 5	Day 6	Day 7
Y / N	Y / N	Y / N	Y / N	Y / N	Y / N	Y / N

Day 8	Day 9	Day 10	Day 11	Day 12	Day 13	Day 14
Y / N	Y / N	Y / N	Y / N	Y / N	Y / N	Y / N

NOTES/QUESTIONS/FEEDBACK:

BODY COMPOSITION PROGRESS:

Starting Weight:	Ending Weight:

Starting BF%:	Ending BF%:

Starting BMI:	Ending BMI:

CIRCUMFERENCE MEASUREMENTS:

	Starting	Ending
Neck		
Bicep		
Chest		
Waist		
Hips		
Thigh		

Million Ways to Live

HEALTHY LIFESTYLE PRINCIPLE: Community

HEALTHY HABIT: Reconnect with Nature

LIFESTYLE TRANSFORMATION PROGRAM

HABIT DETAILS
Reconnecting with nature is therapeutic, relaxing and healing. Get outside and enjoy the outdoors.

TIPS/TRICKS/SUGGESTIONS
- Go on a hike
- Meditate outdoors
- Get some sunshine for a few minutes at lunch
- Go swimming in the ocean or a lake
- Smell flowers
- Climb trees
- Lay on the ground
- Walk barefoot in the sand

HABIT COMPLIANCE: [   ] /14

Day 1	Day 2	Day 3	Day 4	Day 5	Day 6	Day 7
Y / N	Y / N	Y / N	Y / N	Y / N	Y / N	Y / N

Day 8	Day 9	Day 10	Day 11	Day 12	Day 13	Day 14
Y / N	Y / N	Y / N	Y / N	Y / N	Y / N	Y / N

NOTES/QUESTIONS/FEEDBACK:

BODY COMPOSITION PROGRESS:

Starting Weight:

Ending Weight:

Starting BF%:

Ending BF%:

Starting BMI:

Ending BMI:

CIRCUMFERENCE MEASUREMENTS:

	Starting	Ending
Neck		
Bicep		
Chest		
Waist		
Hips		
Thigh		

Healthy Habits Progress & Tracking Sheets

HEALTHY LIFESTYLE PRINCIPLE: Real Food

HEALTHY HABIT: Ditch the Liquid Calories

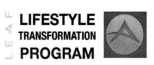

LIFESTYLE TRANSFORMATION PROGRAM

HABIT DETAILS

Drink 2-4 liters of water a day. Unsweetened tea and black coffee are fine too. But **fruit juice, soda, alcohol, sauces, dressings and condiments are out**. Two exceptions post-workout are recovery drinks and fresh green veggie juices.

TIPS/TRICKS/SUGGESTIONS

- Drink Kombucha instead of soda and alcohol
- Use olive oil, balsamic vinegar and fresh-squeezed lemon as dressing
- Don't eat glazed meats - the glaze counts as liquid calories!
- Add Celtic sea salt to water for high-quality minerals and better absorption
- Avoid artificial sweeteners and diet products

HABIT COMPLIANCE: ⬚ /14

Day 1	Day 2	Day 3	Day 4	Day 5	Day 6	Day 7
Y / N	Y / N	Y / N	Y / N	Y / N	Y / N	Y / N

Day 8	Day 9	Day 10	Day 11	Day 12	Day 13	Day 14
Y / N	Y / N	Y / N	Y / N	Y / N	Y / N	Y / N

NOTES/QUESTIONS/FEEDBACK:

BODY COMPOSITION PROGRESS:

Starting Weight:

Ending Weight:

Starting BF%:

Ending BF%:

Starting BMI:

Ending BMI:

CIRCUMFERENCE MEASUREMENTS:

	Starting	Ending
Neck		
Bicep		
Chest		
Waist		
Hips		
Thigh		

Million Ways to Live

HEALTHY LIFESTYLE PRINCIPLE: Lifelong Learning

HEALTHY HABIT: Travel

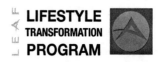

LIFESTYLE TRANSFORMATION PROGRAM

HABIT DETAILS

There is no better way to learn than to travel somewhere new and experience new people, new cultures and new sights. Even if it's only within your city, travel somewhere and experience something new twice.

TIPS/TRICKS/SUGGESTIONS

- Research events and attractions that you've never been to or seen before
- Take a friend with you and enjoy it together
- Try a new cuisine
- Plan an overseas holiday, including setting a budget

HABIT COMPLIANCE: [   ] /2

Trip 1
Y / N

Trip 2
Y / N

NOTES/QUESTIONS/FEEDBACK:

BODY COMPOSITION PROGRESS:

Starting Weight:

Ending Weight:

Starting BF%:

Ending BF%:

Starting BMI:

Ending BMI:

CIRCUMFERENCE MEASUREMENTS:

	Starting	Ending
Neck		
Bicep		
Chest		
Waist		
Hips		
Thigh		

Healthy Habits Progress & Tracking Sheets

HEALTHY LIFESTYLE PRINCIPLE: Rest & Relaxation

HEALTHY HABIT: Muscle Maintenance

LIFESTYLE TRANSFORMATION PROGRAM

HABIT DETAILS

Caring for your muscle tissue will reduce pain, improve recovery, eliminate stress and improve circulation. Whether you get a massage or do it yourself, maintain your muscle tissue at least 20 minutes each day.

TIPS/TRICKS/SUGGESTIONS

- Get a massage
- Do self-massage techniques like foam rolling or ball work
- Get a stretch session

HABIT COMPLIANCE: [   ] /14

Day 1	Day 2	Day 3	Day 4	Day 5	Day 6	Day 7
Y / N	Y / N	Y / N	Y / N	Y / N	Y / N	Y / N

Day 8	Day 9	Day 10	Day 11	Day 12	Day 13	Day 14
Y / N	Y / N	Y / N	Y / N	Y / N	Y / N	Y / N

NOTES/QUESTIONS/FEEDBACK:

BODY COMPOSITION PROGRESS:

Starting Weight:

Ending Weight:

Starting BF%:

Ending BF%:

Starting BMI:

Ending BMI:

CIRCUMFERENCE MEASUREMENTS:

	Starting	Ending
Neck		
Bicep		
Chest		
Waist		
Hips		
Thigh		

Million Ways to Live

HEALTHY LIFESTYLE PRINCIPLE: Community

HEALTHY HABIT: Find Your Cheering Squad

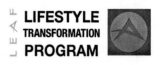

**LIFESTYLE
TRANSFORMATION
PROGRAM**

HABIT DETAILS

Humans are social creatures. Surround yourself with like-minded and healthy people who support you and your goals. Be supportive in return. Everyday, do something to cultivate your sense of community and being more social.

TIPS/TRICKS/SUGGESTIONS

- Eat a meal with friends
- Organize a social event
- Attend a meeting for a like-minded interest group
- Organize a healthy potluck

HABIT COMPLIANCE: [   ] /14

Day 1	Day 2	Day 3	Day 4	Day 5	Day 6	Day 7
Y / N	Y / N	Y / N	Y / N	Y / N	Y / N	Y / N

Day 8	Day 9	Day 10	Day 11	Day 12	Day 13	Day 14
Y / N	Y / N	Y / N	Y / N	Y / N	Y / N	Y / N

NOTES/QUESTIONS/FEEDBACK:

BODY COMPOSITION PROGRESS:

Starting Weight:

Ending Weight:

Starting BF%:

Ending BF%:

Starting BMI:

Ending BMI:

CIRCUMFERENCE MEASUREMENTS:

	Starting	Ending
Neck		
Bicep		
Chest		
Waist		
Hips		
Thigh		

Healthy Habits Progress & Tracking Sheets

HEALTHY LIFESTYLE PRINCIPLE: Love

HEALTHY HABIT: Keep a Gratitude Journal

LIFESTYLE TRANSFORMATION PROGRAM

HABIT DETAILS

Practice gratitude whenever possible, especially when you're frustrated, angry, depressed or disheartened.

TIPS/TRICKS/SUGGESTIONS
- Keep a nightly gratitude log
- Stop arguments with deep breathes and thoughts of gratitude
- Practice gratitude before eating a meal

HABIT COMPLIANCE: [   ] /14

Day 1	Day 2	Day 3	Day 4	Day 5	Day 6	Day 7
Y / N	Y / N	Y / N	Y / N	Y / N	Y / N	Y / N

Day 8	Day 9	Day 10	Day 11	Day 12	Day 13	Day 14
Y / N	Y / N	Y / N	Y / N	Y / N	Y / N	Y / N

NOTES/QUESTIONS/FEEDBACK:

BODY COMPOSITION PROGRESS:

Starting Weight:

Ending Weight:

Starting BF%:

Ending BF%:

Starting BMI:

Ending BMI:

CIRCUMFERENCE MEASUREMENTS:

	Starting	Ending
Neck		
Bicep		
Chest		
Waist		
Hips		
Thigh		

Million Ways to Live

HEALTHY LIFESTYLE PRINCIPLE: Rest & Relaxation

HEALTHY HABIT: The Art of Doing Nothing

L E A F

LIFESTYLE
TRANSFORMATION
PROGRAM

HABIT DETAILS

Learn to cultivate a calm state of mind in the midst of modern day stress and chaos. Meditate for at least 10 minutes every day.

TIPS/TRICKS/SUGGESTIONS

- Focus on your breath
- Count each inhalation and exhalation to 10, then start over
- Don't get mad if your mind wanders - it's normal
- Make sure you're comfortable when you meditate

HABIT COMPLIANCE: [   ] /14

Day 1	Day 2	Day 3	Day 4	Day 5	Day 6	Day 7
Y / N	Y / N	Y / N	Y / N	Y / N	Y / N	Y / N

Day 8	Day 9	Day 10	Day 11	Day 12	Day 13	Day 14
Y / N	Y / N	Y / N	Y / N	Y / N	Y / N	Y / N

NOTES/QUESTIONS/FEEDBACK:

BODY COMPOSITION PROGRESS:

Starting Weight:

Ending Weight:

Starting BF%:

Ending BF%:

Starting BMI:

Ending BMI:

CIRCUMFERENCE MEASUREMENTS:

	Starting	Ending
Neck		
Bicep		
Chest		
Waist		
Hips		
Thigh		

Healthy Habits Progress & Tracking Sheets

WEEK #: 31

HEALTHY LIFESTYLE PRINCIPLE: Lifelong Learning

HEALTHY HABIT: Read Daily

HABIT DETAILS

Whether it's a magazine, self-help book or fiction, read for 20 minutes everyday.

HABIT COMPLIANCE: [   ] /14

Day 1	Day 2	Day 3	Day 4	Day 5	Day 6	Day 7
Y / N	Y / N	Y / N	Y / N	Y / N	Y / N	Y / N

Day 8	Day 9	Day 10	Day 11	Day 12	Day 13	Day 14
Y / N	Y / N	Y / N	Y / N	Y / N	Y / N	Y / N

NOTES/QUESTIONS/FEEDBACK:

BODY COMPOSITION PROGRESS:

Starting Weight:

Ending Weight:

Starting BF%:

Ending BF%:

Starting BMI:

Ending BMI:

CIRCUMFERENCE MEASUREMENTS:

	Starting	Ending
Neck		
Bicep		
Chest		
Waist		
Hips		
Thigh		

219

Million Ways to Live

HEALTHY LIFESTYLE PRINCIPLE: Community

HEALTHY HABIT: Cell Phone Detox

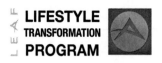
LEAF LIFESTYLE TRANSFORMATION PROGRAM

HABIT DETAILS
Put away your cellphone. Live in the moment and focus on the people and things going on around you when you're out in public or at home with others.

TIPS/TRICKS/SUGGESTIONS
- Turn off your cell phone, don't just put it on silent
- Leave your cell phone in the car when going out to dinner
- Put your cell phone out of reach when in a room with others

HABIT COMPLIANCE: [   ] /14

Day 1	Day 2	Day 3	Day 4	Day 5	Day 6	Day 7
Y / N	Y / N	Y / N	Y / N	Y / N	Y / N	Y / N

Day 8	Day 9	Day 10	Day 11	Day 12	Day 13	Day 14
Y / N	Y / N	Y / N	Y / N	Y / N	Y / N	Y / N

NOTES/QUESTIONS/FEEDBACK:

BODY COMPOSITION PROGRESS:

Starting Weight:

Ending Weight:

Starting BF%:

Ending BF%:

Starting BMI:

Ending BMI:

CIRCUMFERENCE MEASUREMENTS:

	Starting	Ending
Neck		
Bicep		
Chest		
Waist		
Hips		
Thigh		

220

Healthy Habits Progress & Tracking Sheets

WEEK #: 35

HEALTHY LIFESTYLE PRINCIPLE: Lifelong Learning

HEALTHY HABIT: Television Detox

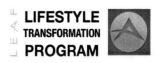

LIFESTYLE TRANSFORMATION PROGRAM

HABIT DETAILS

Turn off your television, and instead invest that time in your friends and family, reading a book, learning new hobbies, getting outside or meditating.

TIPS/TRICKS/SUGGESTIONS

- Try reading instead of watching TV
- Spend time with family and friends
- Call old friends or family members to hear about their life updates
- Start a new hobby like cooking or gardening

HABIT COMPLIANCE: [   ] /14

Day 1	Day 2	Day 3	Day 4	Day 5	Day 6	Day 7
Y / N	Y / N	Y / N	Y / N	Y / N	Y / N	Y / N

Day 8	Day 9	Day 10	Day 11	Day 12	Day 13	Day 14
Y / N	Y / N	Y / N	Y / N	Y / N	Y / N	Y / N

NOTES/QUESTIONS/FEEDBACK:

BODY COMPOSITION PROGRESS:

Starting Weight:

Ending Weight:

Starting BF%:

Ending BF%:

Starting BMI:

Ending BMI:

CIRCUMFERENCE MEASUREMENTS:

	Starting	Ending
Neck		
Bicep		
Chest		
Waist		
Hips		
Thigh		

Million Ways to Live

HEALTHY LIFESTYLE PRINCIPLE: Love

HEALTHY HABIT: Connect Physically

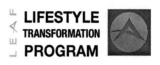

LIFESTYLE TRANSFORMATION PROGRAM

HABIT DETAILS

Physical connection is therapeutic and restorative. Learn to burst your personal bubble.

TIPS/TRICKS/SUGGESTIONS

- Cuddle more often
- Hug someone (if it's a stranger, make sure they're OK with it!)
- Have sex

HABIT COMPLIANCE: [   ] /14

Day 1	Day 2	Day 3	Day 4	Day 5	Day 6	Day 7
Y / N	Y / N	Y / N	Y / N	Y / N	Y / N	Y / N

Day 8	Day 9	Day 10	Day 11	Day 12	Day 13	Day 14
Y / N	Y / N	Y / N	Y / N	Y / N	Y / N	Y / N

NOTES/QUESTIONS/FEEDBACK:

BODY COMPOSITION PROGRESS:

Starting Weight:

Ending Weight:

Starting BF%:

Ending BF%:

Starting BMI:

Ending BMI:

CIRCUMFERENCE MEASUREMENTS:

	Starting	Ending
Neck		
Bicep		
Chest		
Waist		
Hips		
Thigh		

Healthy Habits Progress & Tracking Sheets

HEALTHY LIFESTYLE PRINCIPLE: Real Food

HEALTHY HABIT: Reconnect with the Food Experience

**LIFESTYLE
TRANSFORMATION
PROGRAM**

HABIT DETAILS
Reconnect with the food experience by cooking your own meals, cooking for others, sharing your meals, eating with gratitude, befriending your local farmer or growing your own food.

TIPS/TRICKS/SUGGESTIONS
- Plant herbs for a small home garden
- Visit the local Farmer's Market and forge a relationship with your farmer
- Cook a meal for someone
- Express gratitude before eating

HABIT COMPLIANCE: [   ] /14

Day 1	Day 2	Day 3	Day 4	Day 5	Day 6	Day 7
Y / N	Y / N	Y / N	Y / N	Y / N	Y / N	Y / N

Day 8	Day 9	Day 10	Day 11	Day 12	Day 13	Day 14
Y / N	Y / N	Y / N	Y / N	Y / N	Y / N	Y / N

NOTES/QUESTIONS/FEEDBACK:

BODY COMPOSITION PROGRESS:

Starting Weight:	Ending Weight:

Starting BF%:	Ending BF%:

Starting BMI:	Ending BMI:

CIRCUMFERENCE MEASUREMENTS:

	Starting	Ending
Neck		
Bicep		
Chest		
Waist		
Hips		
Thigh		

223

Million Ways to Live

WEEK #: 41

HEALTHY LIFESTYLE PRINCIPLE: Lifelong Learning

HEALTHY HABIT: Continued Education

**LIFESTYLE
TRANSFORMATION
PROGRAM**

HABIT DETAILS

Whether it's a hobby, a new language, a college course, seminar or lecture, focus on acquiring a new skill or new knowledge. Every day, work towards going deeper and learning more about the subject that you choose.

TIPS/TRICKS/SUGGESTIONS

- Start that hobby you always said you wanted to do
- Try a recreational sport like surfing, rock climbing or paddle boarding
- Enroll in a course or start working towards a certificate

HABIT COMPLIANCE: [   ] /14

Day 1	Day 2	Day 3	Day 4	Day 5	Day 6	Day 7
Y / N	Y / N	Y / N	Y / N	Y / N	Y / N	Y / N

Day 8	Day 9	Day 10	Day 11	Day 12	Day 13	Day 14
Y / N	Y / N	Y / N	Y / N	Y / N	Y / N	Y / N

NOTES/QUESTIONS/FEEDBACK:

BODY COMPOSITION PROGRESS:

Starting Weight:

Ending Weight:

Starting BF%:

Ending BF%:

Starting BMI:

Ending BMI:

CIRCUMFERENCE MEASUREMENTS:

	Starting	Ending
Neck		
Bicep		
Chest		
Waist		
Hips		
Thigh		

Healthy Habits Progress & Tracking Sheets

WEEK #: 43

HEALTHY LIFESTYLE PRINCIPLE: Movement

HEALTHY HABIT: Diversify Exercise

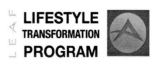
HABIT DETAILS

Diversifying movement is as important as diversifying diet. Try new and different workout modalities for a great brain workout and physical challenge. Diversify 4 - 8 of your workouts.

TIPS/TRICKS/SUGGESTIONS

- Pilates
- Yoga
- Rowing
- Spin

HABIT COMPLIANCE: [   ] /8

Workout 1	Workout 2	Workout 3	Workout 4
Y / N	Y / N	Y / N	Y / N

Workout 5	Workout 6	Workout 7	Workout 8
Y / N	Y / N	Y / N	Y / N

NOTES/QUESTIONS/FEEDBACK:

BODY COMPOSITION PROGRESS:

Starting Weight:	Ending Weight:

Starting BF%:	Ending BF%:

Starting BMI:	Ending BMI:

CIRCUMFERENCE MEASUREMENTS:

	Starting	Ending
Neck		
Bicep		
Chest		
Waist		
Hips		
Thigh		

WEEK #: 45

HEALTHY LIFESTYLE PRINCIPLE:　　Rest & Relaxation

HEALTHY HABIT: Have Fun

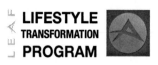

LIFESTYLE TRANSFORMATION PROGRAM

HABIT DETAILS

Schedule four fun activities you've always wanted to do but have been delaying. Can't think of any? Ask friends and tag along for their fun adventures.

TIPS/TRICKS/SUGGESTIONS

- Look up local events and attractions online
- Pick one day and just say yes to any and all requests made of your time by friends and family
- Remember something you used to love doing but don't do any more, and do it

HABIT COMPLIANCE: ☐ /4

Event 1	Event 2	Event 3	Event 4
Y / N	Y / N	Y / N	Y / N

NOTES/QUESTIONS/FEEDBACK:

BODY COMPOSITION PROGRESS:

Starting Weight: ☐　　　**Ending Weight:** ☐

Starting BF%: ☐　　　**Ending BF%:** ☐

Starting BMI: ☐　　　**Ending BMI:** ☐

CIRCUMFERENCE MEASUREMENTS:

	Starting	Ending
Neck		
Bicep		
Chest		
Waist		
Hips		
Thigh		

Healthy Habits Progress & Tracking Sheets

HEALTHY LIFESTYLE PRINCIPLE: Love

HEALTHY HABIT: Date Night

LIFESTYLE TRANSFORMATION PROGRAM

HABIT DETAILS

Reward yourself and spend time with yourself. Alone. Twice.

TIPS/TRICKS/SUGGESTIONS

- Book a massage
- Go to a movie
- Take a stroll along the beach
- Take yourself out for coffee

HABIT COMPLIANCE: [   ] /2

Date 1	Date 2
Y / N	Y / N

NOTES/QUESTIONS/FEEDBACK:

BODY COMPOSITION PROGRESS:

Starting Weight:	Ending Weight:

Starting BF%:	Ending BF%:

Starting BMI:	Ending BMI:

CIRCUMFERENCE MEASUREMENTS:

	Starting	Ending
Neck		
Bicep		
Chest		
Waist		
Hips		
Thigh		

Million Ways to Live

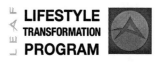

HABIT DETAILS

Practice random acts of kindness with others. Give, and don't expect anything in return.

TIPS/TRICKS/SUGGESTIONS

- Hold a door open for someone
- Buy a stranger a coffee
- Smile at a stranger
- Donate to a charity or cause
- Help a friend in need of advice, support or listening

HABIT COMPLIANCE: [   ] /14

Day 1	Day 2	Day 3	Day 4	Day 5	Day 6	Day 7
Y / N	Y / N	Y / N	Y / N	Y / N	Y / N	Y / N

Day 8	Day 9	Day 10	Day 11	Day 12	Day 13	Day 14
Y / N	Y / N	Y / N	Y / N	Y / N	Y / N	Y / N

NOTES/QUESTIONS/FEEDBACK:

BODY COMPOSITION PROGRESS:

Starting Weight:	Ending Weight:

Starting BF%:	Ending BF%:

Starting BMI:	Ending BMI:

CIRCUMFERENCE MEASUREMENTS:

	Starting	Ending
Neck		
Bicep		
Chest		
Waist		
Hips		
Thigh		

228

Healthy Habits Progress & Tracking Sheets

WEEK #: 51

HEALTHY LIFESTYLE PRINCIPLE:　　Rest & Relaxation

HEALTHY HABIT: Simplify. Simplify. Simplify.

LIFESTYLE TRANSFORMATION PROGRAM

HABIT DETAILS

Declutter your life. The more you have, the more you stress. Remove the superfluous and simplify 4 - 8 areas of your life.

TIPS/TRICKS/SUGGESTIONS

- Clean out and organize your inbox
- Organize your work desk
- Leave destructive relationships or friendships
- Create a 'get out of debt' plan, then do it!

- Have a garage sale
- Throw away old clothes
- Clean your house
- Reconcile your bank accounts

HABIT COMPLIANCE: [   ] /8

Simplification 1	Simplification 2	Simplification 3	Simplification 4
Y / N	Y / N	Y / N	Y / N

Simplification 5	Simplification 6	Simplification 7	Simplification 8
Y / N	Y / N	Y / N	Y / N

NOTES/QUESTIONS/FEEDBACK:

BODY COMPOSITION PROGRESS:

Starting Weight:　　　　Ending Weight:

Starting BF%:　　　　Ending BF%:

Starting BMI:　　　　Ending BMI:

CIRCUMFERENCE MEASUREMENTS:

	Starting	Ending
Neck		
Bicep		
Chest		
Waist		
Hips		
Thigh		

Notes

Introduction: Meet David

[1] Malnick SD, Knobler H. (2006) The medical complications of obesity. QJM. 99(9): 565-579.

[2] Curry SJ, Byers T, Hewitt M, Eds. Fulfilling the Potential for Cancer Prevention and Early Detection. National Cancer Policy Board. Institute of Medicine. National Research Council of the National Academies. Washington, D.C.: National Academies Press, 2003.

[3] Garrison, RJ, et al. (1987) Incidence and precursors of hypertension in young adults: The Framingham Offspring Study, Prev Med. 16: 235-25.

[4] Al-Hazzaa, Hazzaa M., et al. "Lifestyle Factors Associated With Overweight And Obesity Among Saudi Adolescents." BMC Public Health 12.1 (2012): 354-364.

[5] Fast Stats. "Obesity and Overweight". Centers for Disease Control and Prevention. CDC National Center for Health Statistics. November 21, 2013.

[6] Gunta, Sujana, and Robert Mak. "Is Obesity A Risk Factor For

Chronic Kidney Disease In Children?." Pediatric Nephrology 28.10 (2013): 1949-1956.

[7] University of Oxford. "Moderate Obesity Takes Years Off Life Expectancy." ScienceDaily, 20 Mar. 2009.

[8] Goonasegaran AR, "Comparison of the effectiveness of body mass index and body fat percentage in defining body composition." Singapore Medical Journal. 2012 Jun;53(6):403-8.

[9] Srikanthan, Preethi, and Arun S. Karlamangla. "Muscle Mass Index As A Predictor Of Longevity In Older Adults." American Journal Of Medicine 127.6 (2014): 547-553. Academic Search Complete. Web. 17 June 2014.

[10] Grujic, Vera, et al. "Association Between Obesity And Socioeconomic Factors And Lifestyle." Vojnosanitetski Pregled: Military Medical & Pharmaceutical Journal Of Serbia & Montenegro 66.9 (2009): 705-710.

[11] Mietus-Snyder, Michele L., and Robert H. Lustig. "Childhood Obesity: Adrift In The "Limbic Triangle." Annual Review Of Medicine 59.1 (2008): 147-162.

[12] Dyson, P. A. "The Therapeutics Of Lifestyle Management On Obesity." Diabetes, Obesity & Metabolism 12.11 (2010): 941-946.

[13] Temelkova-Kurktschiev, T., and T. S. Stefanov. "Lifestyle And Genetics In Obesity And Type 2 Diabetes." Experimental & Clinical Endocrinology & Diabetes 120.1 (2012): 1-6.

[14] Ford, Jessica, Melanie Spallek, and Annette Dobson. "Self-Rated Health And A Healthy Lifestyle Are The Most Important Predictors Of Survival In Elderly Women." Age & Ageing 37.2

(2008): 194-200.

[15] "Staying Active And Social Prolongs Life Even After 75." Tufts University Health & Nutrition Letter 30.10 (2012): 3.

Real Food

[1] Lessa, N. M. V., et al. "Deposition Of Trans Fatty Acid From Industrial Sources And Its Effect On Different Growth Phases In Rats." Annals Of Nutrition & Metabolism 57.1 (2010): 23-34.

[2] Laake, I et al "A prospective study of intake of trans-fatty acids from ruminant fat, partially hydrogenated vegetable oils, and marine oils and mortality from CVD. The British Journal of Nutrition 2012 Aug;108(4):743-54. doi: 10.1017/S0007114511005897.

[3] Tardy, Anne-Laure, et al. "Ruminant And Industrial Sources Of Trans-Fat And Cardiovascular And Diabetic Diseases." Nutrition Research Reviews24.1 (2011): 111-117.

[4] Mozaffarian, D., et al. "Consumption Of Trans Fats And Estimated Effects On Coronary Heart Disease In Iran." European Journal Of Clinical Nutrition 61.8 (2007): 1004-1010.

[5] Wang, Ye, M. Miriam Jacome-Sosa, and Spencer D. Proctor. "The Role Of Ruminant Trans Fat As A Potential Nutraceutical In The Prevention Of Cardiovascular Disease." Food Research International 46.2 (2012): 460-468.

[6] Eunyong, Cho, et al. "Dairy Foods, Calcium, And Colorectal Cancer: A Pooled Analysis Of 10 Cohort Studies." JNCI: Journal Of The National Cancer Institute 96.13 (2004): 1015-1022.

[7] Ravnskov, U. "The questionable role of saturated and polyunsaturated fatty acids in cardiovascular disease." Journal of

Clinical Epidemiology 1998 Jun;51(6):443-60.

[8] Dong, JY et al. "Dairy consumption and risk of breast cancer: a meta-analysis of prospective cohort studies. Breast Cancer Research and Treatment. 2011 May;127(1):23-31. doi: 10.1007/s10549-011-1467-5.

[9] Cong, Wei-na, et al. "Long-Term Artificial Sweetener Acesulfame Potassium Treatment Alters Neurometabolic Functions In C57BL/6J Mice." Plos ONE 8.8 (2013): 1-18.

[10] Gupta, Sourab, et al. "Artificial Sweeteners." JK Science 14.1 (2012): 2-4.

[11] Soffritti, Morando, et al. "First Experimental Demonstration Of The Multipotential Carcinogenic Effects Of Aspartame Administered In The Feed To Sprague-Dawley Rats." Environmental Health Perspectives 114.3 (2006): 379-385.

[12] Soffritti, Morando, et al. "Life-Span Exposure To Low Doses Of Aspartame Beginning During Prenatal Life Increases Cancer Effects In Rats." Environmental Health Perspectives 115.9 (2007): 1293-1297.

[13] Soffritti, Morando, et al. "Aspartame administered in feed, beginning prenatally through life span, induces cancers of the liver and lung in male Swiss mice." American Journal of Internal Medicine. 2010 Dec;53(12):1197-206. doi: 10.1002/ajim.20896.

[14] Cell Press. "The dark side of artificial sweeteners: Expert reviews negative imact."ScienceDaily, 10 Jul. 2013.

[15] Sara N. Bleich, Julia A. Wolfson, Sienna Vine and Y. Claire Wang. "Diet Beverage Consumption and Caloric Intake Among US Adults Overall and by Body Weight." American Journal of Public Health, January 2014

[16] Bianconi, Eva, et al. "An estimation of the number of cells in the human body." Annals Of Human Biology 40, no. 6 (November 2013): 463-471.

[17] Karam, Jose A. (2009). Apoptosis in Carcinogenesis and Chemotherapy. Netherlands: Springer. ISBN 978-1-4020-9597-9.

[18] Fraser GE, Shavlik DJ. Ten Years of Life: Is It a Matter of Choice?. Arch Intern Med.2001;161(13):1645-1652. doi:10.1001/archinte.161.13.1645.

[19] Mozaffarian, D., et al. "Consumption Of Trans Fats And Estimated Effects On Coronary Heart Disease In Iran." European Journal Of Clinical Nutrition 61.8 (2007): 1004-1010.

[20] Cozma AI, Sievenpiper JL, de Souza RJ et al. "Effect of fructose on glycemic control in diabetes: a systematic review and meta-analysis of controlled feeding trials". St Michael's Hospital, Toronto, ON, Canada. Diabetes Care 2012; 35: 1611–20.

[21] Rodriguez-Sierra, JF et al. "Monosodium Glutamate disruption of behavioral and endocrine function in the female rat." Neuroendocrinology 1980; 31:228–235 (DOI:10.1159/000123079)

[22] University of North Carolina at Chapel Hill. "MSG Use Linked To Obesity." ScienceDaily, 14 Aug. 2008.

[23] Luz, Jacqueline, et al. "Effect Of Food Restriction On Energy Expenditure Of Monosodium Glutamate-Induced Obese Rats." Annals Of Nutrition & Metabolism 56.1 (2010): 31-35.

[24] Masic, Una, et al. "Does Monosodium Glutamate Interact With Macronutrient Composition To Influence Subsequent Appetite?." Physiology & Behavior 116-117.(2013): 23-29.

[25] Luscombe-Marsh, ND et al. "The addition of monosodium

glutamate and inosine monophosphate-5 to high-protein meals: effects on satiety, and energy and macronutrient intakes." British Journal of Nutrition. 2009 Sep;102(6):929-37. doi: 10.1017/S0007114509297212.

[26] McLennan, P. L., et al. "The Influence Of Red Meat Intake Upon The Response To A Resistance Exercise-Training Program In Older Australians." Asia Pacific Journal Of Clinical Nutrition 12. (2003): 68.

[27] Biesalski, H.-K. "Meat As A Component Of A Healthy Diet – Are There Any Risks Or Benefits If Meat Is Avoided In The Diet?." Meat Science 70.3 (2005): 509-524.

[28] Do, Ron, et al. "The Effect Of Chromosome 9P21 Variants On Cardiovascular Disease May Be Modified By Dietary Intake: Evidence From A Case/Control And A Prospective Study." Plos Medicine 8.10 (2011): 1-10.

[29] Vadivel, Vellingiri, Catherine N. Kunyanga, and Hans K. Biesalski. "Health Benefits Of Nut Consumption With Special Reference To Body Weight Control." Nutrition 28.11/12 (2012): 1089-1097.

[30] Rein, Maarit J., et al. "Bioavailability Of Bioactive Food Compounds: A Challenging Journey To Bioefficacy." British Journal Of Clinical Pharmacology 75.3 (2013): 588-602.

[31] Torheim, L. E., et al. "Nutrient Adequacy And Dietary Diversity In Rural Mali: Association And Determinants." European Journal Of Clinical Nutrition58.4 (2004): 594-604.

[32] Arimond, Mary, and Marie T. Ruel. "Dietary Diversity Is Associated With Child Nutritional Status: Evidence From 11 Demographic And Health Surveys." Journal Of Nutrition 134.10 (2004): 2579-2585.

[33] Azadbakht, L., P. Mirmiran, and F. Azizi. "Dietary Diversity Score Is Favorably Associated With The Metabolic Syndrome In Tehranian Adults." International Journal Of Obesity 29.11 (2005): 1361-1367.

[34] Bernstein, Melissa, et al. "Higher Dietary Variety Is Associated With Better Nutritional Status In Frail Elderly People." Journal Of The American Dietetic Association 102.8 (2002): 1096-1104.

[35] Fesler, Katie. "The Craving Brain." Tufts Nutrition Magazine. Winter 2014. Extracted from http://now.tufts.edu/articles/craving-brain

[36] Oyinlola Oyebode, Vanessa Gordon-Dseagu, Alice Walker, Jennifer S Mindell.Fruit and vegetable consumption and all-cause, cancer and CVD mortality: analysis of Health Survey for England data. J Epidemiol Community Health, 31 March 2014 DOI: 10.1136/jech-2013-203500

[37] Barrett, Diane. "Maximizing the Nutritional Value of Fruits and Vegetables." Food Technology 61(4):40-44.

[38] Danesi, F., and A. Bordoni. "Effect Of Home Freezing And Italian Style Of Cooking On Antioxidant Activity Of Edible Vegetables." Journal Of Food Science 73.6 (2008): H109-H112.

[39] Bacchiocca M. et al. "Polyphenols and antioxidant capacity of vegetables under fresh and frozen conditions." Istituto di Chimica Biologica, G. Fornaini Università di Urbino, Urbino (PU), Italy. Journal of Agricultural and Food Chemistry, 2003 Apr 9; 51(8): 2222-6

[40] "Don't Give Frozen Produce The Cold Shoulder." Harvard Heart Letter 20.6 (2010): 6.

[41] Nassauer, Sara. "Frozen Produce Seeks Respect Promising

Nutrients, Convenience." Wall Street Journal - Eastern Edition 31 Dec. 2013

[42] Marler, John. "Human Health, the Nutritional Quality of Harvested Food and Sustainable Farming Systems." Nutrition Security Institute. 2006

[43] Reganold, John P., et al. "Fruit And Soil Quality Of Organic And Conventional Strawberry Agroecosystems." Plos ONE 5.9 (2010): 1-14.

[44] Oliveira, Aurelice B., et al. "The Impact Of Organic Farming On Quality Of Tomatoes Is Associated To Increased Oxidative Stress During Fruit Development." Plos ONE 8.2 (2013): 1-6.

[45] Connelly, Patrice. "Feedlot Meat In Australia: Desirable Or Dangerous?." Journal Of The Australian Traditional-Medicine Society 15.1 (2009): 15-17.

[46] Leheska, J. M., et al. "Effects Of Conventional And Grass-Feeding Systems On The Nutrient Composition Of Beef." Journal Of Animal Science86.12 (2008): 3575-3585.

[47] Adeyeye, Emmanuel. "Nutritional Values Of The Lipid Composition Of The Free-Range Chicken Eggs." Agriculture & Biology Journal Of North America 3.9 (2012): 374-384.

[48] "A Generation in Jeopardy: How pesticides are undermining our children's health and intelligence." Pesticide Action Network North America. 2013.

[49] Laetz, CA, DH Baldwin, TK Collier, V Hebert, JD Stark and NL Scholz. 2009. The synergistic toxicity of pesticide mixtures: implications for risk assessment and the conservation of endangered Pacific salmon. Environmental Health Perspectives doi: 10.1289/ehp.0800096.

[50] Carman, Judy. "A long-term toxicology study on pigs fed a combined genetically modified (GM) soy and GM maize diet". Journal of Organic Systems. Vol 8 No. 1 (2013)

[51] Kuiper, H.A., G.A. kleter., H.P.J.M noteborn. And E.J. kok. Assessment of the food safety issues related to genetically modified foods. Plant Journal, 27(6): 503-528 (2001).

[52] de Vendômois JS, Roullier F, Cellier D, Séralini GE. A Comparison of the Effects of Three GM Corn Varieties on Mammalian Health. Int J Biol Sci 2009; 5(7):706-726. doi:10.7150/ijbs.5.706.

[53] Zhang, Lin, et al. "Exogenous plant MIR168a specifically targets mammalian LDLRAP1: evidence of cross-kingdom regulation by microRNA." Cell Research 2012. V22.1: 107 -126

[54] Estimates of Foodborne Illness in the United States. Centers for Disease Control and Prevention. 2011.

[55] Centers for Disease Control and Prevention. "Tracking and Reporting Foodborne Disease Outbreaks." National Center for Emerging and Zoonotic Infectious Diseases, Division of Foodborne, Waterborne, and Environmental Diseases

[56] Zuniga, Krystle, and John W. Erdman Jr. "Tomato, Broccoli, Soy And Reduced Prostate Cancer Risk: Whole Foods Or Their Bioactive Components?." Journal Of Food & Drug Analysis 20.(2012): 280-282.

[57] Clarke, John D., et al. "Bioavailability And Inter-Conversion Of Sulforaphane And Erucin In Human Subjects Consuming Broccoli Sprouts Or Broccoli Supplement In A Cross-Over Study Design." Pharmacological Research 64.5 (2011): 456-463.

[58] Katz, David. "The Case For Natural Foods." Prevention 62.3 (2010): 124-127.

[59] Barr, Sadie B., and Jonathan C. Wright. "Postprandial Energy Expenditure In Whole-Food And Processed-Food Meals: Implications For Daily Energy Expenditure." Food & Nutrition Research 54.(2010): 1-9.

[60] D.L. Katz and S. Meller. "Can We Say What Diet Is Best for Health?" Annual Review of Public Health, Vol. 35: 83 -103 (Volume publication date March 2014)

[61] Cornelius, Marilyn C., et al. "Coffee, CYP1A2 Genotype, And Risk Of Myocardial Infarction." JAMA: Journal Of The American Medical Association295.10 (2006): 1135-1141.

[62] Stubbs, James, et al. "Measuring the difference between actual and reported food intakes in the context of energy balance under laboratory conditions." British Journal of Nutrition / FirstView Article pp 1-12. March 2014

[63] Kong, Angela, et al. "Self-Monitoring And Eating-Related Behaviors Are Associated With 12-Month Weight Loss In Postmenopausal Overweight-To-Obese Women." Journal Of The Academy Of Nutrition & Dietetics 112.9 (2012): 1428-1435.

[64] Li, Liaoliao, Zhi Wang, and Zhiyi Zuo. "Chronic Intermittent Fasting Improves Cognitive Functions And Brain Structures In Mice." Plos ONE 8.6 (2013): 1-7.

[65] Chia-Wei Cheng, et al. "Prolonged Fasting Reduces IGF-1/PKA to Promote Hematopoietic-Stem-Cell-Based Regeneration and Reverse Immunosuppression." Cell Stem Cell, 2014; 14 (6): 810 DOI:10.1016/j.stem.2014.04.014

[66] Gladstone Institutes. "How calorie restriction influences longevity: Protecting cells from damage caused by chronic disease."ScienceDaily, 6 Dec. 2012.

[67] Heilbronn, Leonie K., et al. "Effect Of 6-Month Calorie Restriction On Biomarkers Of Longevity, Metabolic Adaptation, And Oxidative Stress: A Randomized Controlled Trial." JAMA: Journal Of The American Medical Association 295.13 (2006): 1539

[68] Mattison, Julie A., et al. "Impact Of Caloric Restriction On Health And Survival In Rhesus Monkeys From The NIA Study." Nature 489.7415 (2012): 318-321.

[69] Bonjour, JP. "Dietary protein: an essential nutrient for bone health." Journal of the American College of Nutrition. 2005 Dec;24(6 Suppl):526S-36S.

[70] Kerstetter, JE et al. "Dietary protein and skeletal health: a review of recent human research." Current Opinion in Lipidology. 2011 Feb;22(1):16-20. doi: 10.1097/MOL.0b013e3283419441.

[71] Martin, William F., Lawrence E. Armstrong, and Nancy R. Rodriguez. "Dietary Protein Intake And Renal Function." Nutrition & Metabolism 2.(2005): 25-9.

[72] Olivier, R. "Amino Acids, Blood Sugar Balance and Muscle Protein Maintenance." Original Internist 16.3 (2009): 131-138.

[73] Gannon, Mary et al. "Effect of a High-Protein, Low-Carbohydrate Diet on Blood Glucose Control in People With Type 2 Diabetes." Diabetes September 2004vol. 53 no. 9 2375-2382

[74] Pasiakos, Stefan M., et al. "Effects Of High-Protein Diets On Fat-Free Mass And Muscle Protein Synthesis Following Weight Loss: A Randomized Controlled Trial." FASEB Journal 27.9

(2013): 3837-3847.

[75] Santos, F. L., et al. "Systematic Review And Meta-Analysis Of Clinical Trials Of The Effects Of Low Carbohydrate Diets On Cardiovascular Risk Factors." Obesity Reviews 13.11 (2012): 1048-1066.

[76] Hession, M., et al. "Systematic Review Of Randomized Controlled Trials Of Low-Carbohydrate Vs. Low-Fat/Low-Calorie Diets In The Management Of Obesity And Its Comorbidities." Obesity Reviews 10.1 (2009): 36-50.

[77] Mente, Andrew, et al. "A Systematic Review Of The Evidence Supporting A Causal Link Between Dietary Factors And Coronary Heart Disease." Archives Of Internal Medicine 169.7 (2009): 659-669.

[78] Ravnskov, U. "The questionable role of saturated and polyunsaturated fatty acids in cardiovascular disease." Journal of Clinical Epidemiology 1998 Jun; 51(6):443-60.

[79] Siri-Tarino, Patty et al. "Saturated fat, carbohydrate, and cardiovascular disease." The American Journal of Clinical Nutrition March 2010vol. 91 no. 3 502-509

[80] Basciano, Heather, Lisa Federico, and Khosrow Adeli. "Fructose, Insulin Resistance, And Metabolic Dyslipidemia." Nutrition & Metabolism 2.(2005): 5-14.

[81] Stanhope, KL et al. "Adverse metabolic effects of dietary fructose: results from the recent epidemiological, clinical, and mechanistic studies. Current Opinion in Lipidology. 2013 Jun;24(3):198-206. doi: 10.1097/MOL.0b013e3283613bca.

[82] Ludwig, David S, Karen E Peterson, and Steven L Gortmaker. "Relation Between Consumption Of Sugar-Sweetened Drinks And

Childhood Obesity: A Prospective, Observational Analysis." Lancet 357.9255 (2001): 505.

[83] "Sugar-Sweetened Beverages Increase Risk Of Coronary Heart Disease In Women." Nutrition Research Newsletter 28.5. 2009: 8.

[84] Bantle, John P. "Dietary Fructose And Metabolic Syndrome And Diabetes." Journal Of Nutrition 139.6 (2009): 1263S-1268S.

[85] Basu, Sanjay, et al. "The Relationship Of Sugar To Population-Level Diabetes Prevalence: An Econometric Analysis Of Repeated Cross-Sectional Data." Plos ONE 8.2 (2013): 1-8.

[86] Page, Kathleen A., et al. "Effects Of Fructose Vs Glucose On Regional Cerebral Blood Flow In Brain Regions Involved With Appetite And Reward Pathways." JAMA: Journal Of The American Medical Association 309.1 (2013): 63-70.

[87] Kerrie A. Hert, Paul S. Fisk, Yeong S. Rhee, Ardith R. Brunt. "Decreased consumption of sugar-sweetened beverages improved selected biomarkers of chronic disease risk among us adults: 1999 to 2010". Nutrition Research - 14 November 2013 (10.1016/j.nutres.2013.10.005)

[88] De Koning, Lawrence, et al. "Sweetened Beverage Consumption, Incident Coronary Heart Disease, And Biomarkers Of Risk In Men." Circulation125.14 (2012): 1735-1741.

[89] Kosova, Ethan C., Peggy Auinger, and Andrew A. Bremer. "The Relationships Between Sugar-Sweetened Beverage Intake And Cardiometabolic Markers In Young Children." Journal Of The Academy Of Nutrition & Dietetics 113.2 (2013): 219-227.

[90] Rauzon, Suzanne et al. "An evaluation of the school lunch initiative." Center for Weight and Health, University of California at Berkeley. 2010.

[91] David A. Shoham, Liping Tong, Peter J. Lamberson, Amy H. Auchincloss, Jun Zhang, Lara Dugas, Jay S. Kaufman, Richard S. Cooper, Amy Luke. An Actor-Based Model of Social Network Influence on Adolescent Body Size, Screen Time, and Playing Sports. PLoS ONE, 2012; 7 (6): e39795

[92] Christakis, Nicholas A., and James H. Fowler. "The Spread Of Obesity In A Large Social Network Over 32 Years." New England Journal Of Medicine 357.4 (2007): 370-379.

[93] Macht, Michael. "How Emotions Affect Eating: A Five-Way Model." Appetite 50.1 (2008): 1-11.

[94] Emmons, Robert A., and Michael E. McCullough. "Counting Blessings Versus Burdens: An Experimental Investigation Of Gratitude And Subjective Well-Being In Daily Life." Journal Of Personality & Social Psychology 84.2 (2003): 377-389.

[95] Tramullas, Mónica, Timothy G. Dinan, and John F. Cryan. "Chronic Psychosocial Stress Induces Visceral Hyperalgesia In Mice." Stress: The International Journal On The Biology Of Stress 15.3 (2012): 281-292.

[96] Mönnikes H., "Role of Stress in Functional Gastrointestinal Disorders. Evidence for Stress-Induced Alterations in Gastrointestinal Motility and Sensitivity." Digestive Diseases. Vol. 19, No. 3, 2001.

Movement

[1] Prostyakov, I., B. Morukov, and I. Morukov. "Changes In Bone Mineral Density And Microarchitecture In Cosmonauts After A Six-Month Space Flight." Human Physiology 38.7 (2012): 727-731.

[2] Bogdanis, Gregory C. "Effects Of Physical Activity And

Inactivity On Muscle Fatigue." Frontiers In Physiology 3. (2012): 1-15.

[3] Beach, Tyson A.C., et al. "Effects Of Prolonged Sitting On The Passive Flexion Stiffness Of The In Vivo Lumbar Spine." Spine Journal 5.2 (2005): 145-154.

[4] Hamilton, Marc T., Deborah G. Hamilton, and Theodore W. Zderic. "Role Of Low Energy Expenditure And Sitting In Obesity, Metabolic Syndrome, Type 2 Diabetes, And Cardiovascular Disease." Diabetes 56.11 (2007): 2655-2667.

[5] Warren, Tatiana Y., et al. "Sedentary Behaviors Increase Risk Of Cardiovascular Disease Mortality In Men." Medicine & Science In Sports & Exercise 42.5 (2010): 879-885.

[6] Bjørk Petersen, Christina, et al. "Total Sitting Time And Risk Of Myocardial Infarction, Coronary Heart Disease And All-Cause Mortality In A Prospective Cohort Of Danish Adults." International Journal Of Behavioral Nutrition & Physical Activity 11.1 (2014): 1-22.

[7] Terra, R., et al. "Exercise Improves The Th1 Response By Modulating Cytokine And NO Production In BALB/C Mice." International Journal Of Sports Medicine 34.7 (2013): 661-666.

[8] Chaput, Jean-Philippe, et al. "Combined Associations Between Moderate To Vigorous Physical Activity And Sedentary Behaviour With Cardiometabolic Risk Factors In Children." Applied Physiology, Nutrition & Metabolism 38.5 (2013): 477-483.

[9] Jones, Simon. "Endurance Exercise, The Fountain Of Youth, And The Mitochondrial Key." UBC Medical Journal 3.1 (2011): 26-27.

[10] Goldman, Robert. "Exercise -- The Ultimate Anti-Aging

Pill." Total Health 20.3 (1998): 11.

[11] Bentsen, Signe Berit, et al. "Anxiety And Depression Following Pulmonary Rehabilitation." Scandinavian Journal Of Caring Sciences 27.3 (2013): 541-550.

[12] Danielsson, Louise, et al. "Exercise In The Treatment Of Major Depression: A Systematic Review Grading The Quality Of Evidence." Physiotherapy Theory & Practice 29.8 (2013): 573-585.

[13] MacIntosh, Bradley J., et al. "Impact Of A Single Bout Of Aerobic Exercise On Regional Brain Perfusion And Activation Responses In Healthy Young Adults." Plos ONE 9.1 (2014): 1-7.

[14] T. J. Schoenfeld, P. Rada, P. R. Pieruzzini, B. Hsueh, E. Gould. "Physical Exercise Prevents Stress-Induced Activation of Granule Neurons and Enhances Local Inhibitory Mechanisms in the Dentate Gyrus." *Journal of Neuroscience*, 2013; 33 (18): 7770 DOI: 10.1523/JNEUROSCI.5352-12.2013

[15] Benjamin N. Greenwood, Katie G. Spence, Danielle M. Crevling, Peter J. Clark, Wendy C. Craig, Monika Fleshner. "Exercise-induced stress resistance is independent of exercise controllability and the medial prefrontal cortex." *European Journal of Neuroscience*, 2013; 37 (3): 469 DOI: 10.1111/ejn.12044

[16] Fonseca, Hélder, et al. "Bone Quality: The Determinants Of Bone Strength And Fragility." Sports Medicine 44.1 (2014): 37-53.

[17] Shephard, Roy J., et al. "Objectively Measured Physical Activity And Progressive Loss Of Lean Tissue In Older Japanese Adults: Longitudinal Data From The Nakanojo Study." Journal Of The American Geriatrics Society 61.11 (2013): 1887-1893.

[18] Bolam, K. A., J. G. Z. van Uffelen, and D. R. Taaffe. "The Effect Of Physical Exercise On Bone Density In Middle-Aged And Older Men: A Systematic Review." Osteoporosis International 24.11 (2013): 2749-2762.

[19] Marques, Elisa, Jorge Mota, and Joana Carvalho. "Exercise Effects On Bone Mineral Density In Older Adults: A Meta-Analysis Of Randomized Controlled Trials." Age 34.6 (2012): 1493-1515.

[20] University of Washington. "Digestive Problems May Impede Overweight People From Exercising." ScienceDaily. ScienceDaily, 8 December 2005.

[21] Lane, Kirstin, Dan Worsley, and Don McKenzie. "Exercise And The Lymphatic System: Implications For Breast-Cancer Survivors." Sports Medicine 35.6 (2005): 461-471.

[22] Gracovetsky, Serge. "The Spinal Engine." Springer-Verlag; 1st edition (March 1989)

[23] Chang, Young-Hui et al. "The independent effects of gravity and inertia on running mechanics." The Journal of Experimental Biology 203, 229–238 (2000)

[24] Levin, Stephen M. "The Tensegrity-Truss As A Model For Spine Mechanics: Biotensegrity." Journal Of Mechanics In Medicine & Biology2.3/4 (2002): 375.

[25] Schick, Evan, et al. "A Comparison Of Muscle Activation Between A Smith Machine And Free Weight Bench Press." Journal Of Strength & Conditioning Research (Lippincott Williams & Wilkins) 24.3 (2010): 779-784.

[26] Junghoon, Kim, et al. "Objectively Measured Light-Intensity Lifestyle Activity And Sedentary Time Are Independently

Associated With Metabolic Syndrome: A Cross-Sectional Study Of Japanese Adults." International Journal Of Behavioral Nutrition & Physical Activity 10.1 (2013): 30-36.

[27] Fortes, Cristina, et al. "Walking Four Times Weekly For At Least 15 Min Is Associated With Longevity In A Cohort Of Very Elderly People."Maturitas 74.3 (2013): 246-251.

[28] Kazuki, Fujita et al. "Walking and Mortality in Japan: The Miyagi Cohort Study." Journal of Epidemiology. 2004 Feb;14 Suppl 1:S26-32.

[29] Saunders, Travis John, et al. "Associations Of Sedentary Behavior, Sedentary Bouts And Breaks In Sedentary Time With Cardiometabolic Risk In Children With A Family History Of Obesity." Plos ONE 8.11 (2013): 1-9.

[30] Williams, Paul "Greater Weight Loss From Running Than Walking During A 6.2-Yr Prospective Follow-Up." Medicine & Science In Sports & Exercise 45.4 (2013): 706-713.

[31] Fogelholm, Mikael. "Walking For The Management Of Obesity." Disease Management & Health Outcomes 13.1 (2005): 9-18.

[32] Hardy, Susan E., et al. "Improvement In Usual Gait Speed Predicts Better Survival In Older Adults." Journal Of The American Geriatrics Society 55.11 (2007): 1727-1734.

[33] Studenski, Stephanie, et al. "Gait Speed And Survival In Older Adults." JAMA: Journal Of The American Medical Association 305.1 (2011): 50-58.

[34] Lee, Duck-chul, et al. "Review: Mortality Trends In The General Population: The Importance Of Cardiorespiratory Fitness." Journal Of Psychopharmacology 24.S4 (2010): 27-35.

[35] Boutcher, Stephen H. "High-Intensity Intermittent Exercise And Fat Loss." Journal Of Obesity (2011): 1-10.

[36] "Effects Of High-Intensity Exercise Training On Body Composition, Abdominal Fat Loss, And Cardiorespiratory Fitness In Middle-Aged Korean Females." Applied Physiology, Nutrition & Metabolism 37.6 (2012): 1019-1027.

[37] Salvadori, Alberto, et al. "Short Bouts Of Anaerobic Exercise Increase Non-Esterified Fatty Acids Release In Obesity." European Journal Of Nutrition 53.1 (2014): 243-249.

[38] Pacey, Verity, et al. "Generalized Joint Hypermobility And Risk Of Lower Limb Joint Injury During Sport." American Journal Of Sports Medicine 38.7 (2010): 1487-1497.

[39] McQuade, KJ. "A Case-Control Study of Running Injuries: Comparison of Patterns-of Runners With and Without Running Injuries." The Journal of Orthopaedic and Sports Physical Therapy. 1986;8(2):81-4.

[40] DiFiori, John P., et al. "Overuse Injuries And Burnout In Youth Sports: A Position Statement From The American Medical Society For Sports Medicine." Clinical Journal Of Sport Medicine 24.1 (2014): 3-20.

[41] Wilder, RP et al. "Overuse injuries: tendinopathies, stress fractures, compartment syndrome, and shin splints." Clinical Sports Medicine. 2004 Jan;23(1):55-81, vi.

[42] Macintyre, J.G. et al. "Running Injuries: A Clinical Study of 4,173 Cases." Clinical Journal of Sport Medicine. April 1991. Volume 1. Issue 2.

[43] Chang, Young-Hui, and Hsuan-Wen Cathy Huang. "The Independent Effects Of Gravity And Inertia On Running

Mechanics." Journal Of Experimental Biology 203.2 (2000): 229.

[44] Shors, T.J., et al. "Use It Or Lose It: How Neurogenesis Keeps The Brain Fit For Learning." Behavioural Brain Research 227.2 (2012): 450-458.

[45] Helen J Huang, Alaa A Ahmed. "Older adults learn less, but still reduce metabolic cost, during motor adaptation." Journal of NeurophysiologyOct 2013,DOI: 10.1152/jn.00401.2013

[46] Sparrow, William A., et al. "Aging Effects On The Metabolic And Cognitive Energy Cost Of Interlimb Coordination." Journals Of Gerontology Series A: Biological Sciences & Medical Sciences 60A.3 (2005): 312-319.

Rest & Relaxation

[1] Crosby, Karen M., et al. "Endocannabinoids Gate State-Dependent Plasticity Of Synaptic Inhibition In Feeding Circuits." Neuron 71.3 (2011): 529-541.

[2] Cohen, Sheldon, et al. "Chronic Stress, Glucocorticoid Receptor Resistance, Inflammation, And Disease Risk." Proceedings Of The National Academy Of Sciences Of The United States Of America 109.16 (2012): 5995-5999.

[3] Yuen, Eunice Y., et al. "Repeated Stress Causes Cognitive Impairment By Suppressing Glutamate Receptor Expression And Function In Prefrontal Cortex." Neuron 73.5 (2012): 962-977.

[4] Mather, Mara, and Nichole R. Lighthall. "Risk And Reward Are Processed Differently In Decisions Made Under Stress." Current Directions In Psychological Science (Sage Publications Inc.) 21.1 (2012): 36-41.

[5] Bhasin, Manoj K., et al. "Relaxation Response Induces Temporal

Transcriptome Changes In Energy Metabolism, Insulin Secretion And Inflammatory Pathways." Plos ONE 8.5 (2013): 1-13.

[6] Jen-Chen, Tsai, et al. "The Beneficial Effects Of Tai Chi Chuan On Blood Pressure And Lipid Profile And Anxiety Status In A Randomized Controlled Trial." Journal Of Alternative & Complementary Medicine 9.5 (2003): 747-754.

[7] Sebastian M Schmid, Manfred Hallschmid, Prof Bernd Schultes. The metabolic burden of sleep loss. *The Lancet Diabetes & Endocrinology*, March 2014 DOI:10.1016/S2213-8587(14)70012-9

[8] Croft, Janet B., et al. "Association Between Perceived Insufficient Sleep, Frequent Mental Distress, Obesity And Chronic Diseases Among US Adults, 2009 Behavioral Risk Factor Surveillance System." BMC Public Health 13.1 (2013): 1-8.

[9] Killgore WD. "Effects of sleep deprivation on cognition." Progress in Brain Research. 2010;185:105-29. doi: 10.1016/B978-0-444-53702-7.00007-5.

[10] Benedict C et al. Acute sleep deprivation increases serum levels of neuron-specific enolase (NSE) and S100 calcium binding protein B (S-100B) in healthy young men. SLEEP, December 2013

[11] L. Xie, H. Kang, Q. Xu, M. J. Chen, Y. Liao, M. Thiyagarajan, J. O'Donnell, D. J. Christensen, C. Nicholson, J. J. Iliff, T. Takano, R. Deane, M. Nedergaard. Sleep Drives Metabolite Clearance from the Adult Brain. *Science*, 2013; 342 (6156): 373 DOI: 10.1126/science.1241224

[12] Hoevenaar-Blom M, Spijkerman AMW, Kromhout D, Verschuren WMM. Sufficient sleep duration contributes to lower cardiovascular disease risk in addition to four traditional lifestyle factors: the MORGEN study. *Eur J Prevent Cardiol*, 2013

DOI: 10.1177/2047487313493057

[13] University of Colorado at Boulder. "Nap-deprived tots may be missing out on more than sleep." ScienceDaily. ScienceDaily, 21 January 2012.

[14] University of California - Berkeley. "Midday nap markedly boosts the brain's learning capacity." ScienceDaily. ScienceDaily, 22 February 2010.

[15] Skinner, Natalie, and Neil Brewer. "The Dynamics Of Threat And Challenge Appraisals Prior To Stressful Achievement Events." Journal Of Personality & Social Psychology 83.3 (2002): 678-692.

[16] J. D. Crane, D. I. Ogborn, C. Cupido, S. Melov, A. Hubbard, J. M. Bourgeois, M. A. Tarnopolsky, Massage Therapy Attenuates Inflammatory Signaling After Exercise-Induced Muscle Damage. Sci. Transl. Med. 4, 119ra13 (2012).

[17] Pressman, SD. Et al. "Association of Enjoyable Leisure Activities with Psychological and Physical Well-being." Psychosomatic Medicine. 71:7 (2009): 725-732

Lifelong Learning

[1] Arnas, Yaşare Aktaş. "The Effects Of Television Food Advertisement On Children's Food Purchasing Requests." Pediatrics International 48.2 (2006): 138-145.

[2] Lisa Powell et al. "Nutritional Content of Food and Beverage Products in Television Advertisements Seen on Children's Programming." Childhood Obesity, December 2013.

[3] University of Gothenburg. "High-calorie, low-nutrient foods in kids' TV programs." ScienceDaily. ScienceDaily, 23 April 2014.

[4] Miller, Sonia A., et al. "Association Between Television Viewing And Poor Diet Quality In Young Children." International Journal Of Pediatric Obesity 3.3 (2008): 168-176.

[5] Elmore, Tim. "Left Brain Schools in a Right Brain World." Growing Leaders. 2009.

[6] Sir Ken Robinson. RSA Animate – Changing Education Paradigms. 2010. Viewable at http://www.npr.org/blogs/thetwo-way/2013/12/03/248329823/u-s-high-school-students-slide-in-math-reading-science

[7] Chappell, Bill. "US students slide in global ranking on math, reading, science." NPR. December 3, 2013. Extracted from http://www.npr.org/blogs/thetwo-way/2013/12/03/248329823/u-s-high-school-students-slide-in-math-reading-science

[8] Chiron, C. et.al. "The right brain hemisphere is dominant in human infants." Brain: A Journal of Neurology 120.6 (1997): 1057-1065.

[9] Porter, Benjamin. "Learning New Skills Keeps an Aging Mind Sharp." Association for Psychological Science, 21 October 2013.

[10] Wilson, Robert et al. "Life-span cognitive activity, neuropathologic burden, and cognitive aging." Neurology July 23, 2013 vol. 81 no. 4 314-321

[11] Park, Denise C., et al. "The Impact Of Sustained Engagement On Cognitive Function In Older Adults: The Synapse Project." Psychological Science (Sage Publications Inc.) 25.1 (2014): 103-112.

[12] "Reading can help reduce stress". The Telegraph. March 30,

2009.

[13] Friedland, Robert P., et al. "Patients With Alzheimer's Disease Have Reduced Activities In Midlife Compared With Healthy.." Proceedings Of The National Academy Of Sciences Of The United States Of America 98.6 (2001): 3440.

[14] Bower, Peter, et al. "Influence Of Initial Severity Of Depression On Effectiveness Of Low Intensity Interventions: Meta-Analysis Of Individual Patient Data." BMJ: British Medical Journal 346.7899 (2013): 12.

[15] Williams, Chris, et al. "Guided Self-Help Cognitive Behavioural Therapy For Depression In Primary Care: A Randomised Controlled Trial."Plos Clinical Trials 8.1 (2013): 1-7.

[16] Bal, P. Matthijs, and Martijn Veltkamp. "How Does Fiction Reading Influence Empathy? An Experimental Investigation On The Role Of Emotional Transportation." Plos ONE 8.1 (2013): 1-12.

[17] Comer Kidd, David, and Emanuele Castano. "Reading Literary Fiction Improves Theory Of Mind." Science 342.6156 (2013): 377-380.

[18] Pinto Pereira, Snehal M., Myung Ki, and Chris Power. "Sedentary Behaviour And Biomarkers For Cardiovascular Disease And Diabetes In Mid-Life: The Role Of Television-Viewing And Sitting At Work." Plos ONE 7.2 (2012): 1-9.

[19] Kim, Yeonju, et al. "Association Between Various Sedentary Behaviours And All-Cause, Cardiovascular Disease And Cancer Mortality: The Multiethnic Cohort Study." International Journal Of Epidemiology 42.4 (2013): 1040-1056.

[20] American College of Cardiology. "TV linked to poor snacking habits, cardiovascular risk in middle schoolers." ScienceDaily. ScienceDaily, 28 March 2014.

[21] Lindsay A. Robertson, et al. Childhood and Adolescent Television Viewing and Antisocial Behavior in Early Adulthood. Pediatrics, February 18, 2013.

[22] Amy I. Nathanson, et al. The Relation Between Television Exposure and Theory of Mind Among Preschoolers. Journal of Communication, November 2013.

[23] Lear, Scott A., et al. The association between ownership of common household devices and obesity and diabetes in high, middle and low income countries. Canadian Medical Association Journal, 2014

[24] Veerman, J. Lennert, et al. "Television Viewing Time And Reduced Life Expectancy: A Life Table Analysis." British Journal Of Sports Medicine. 46.13 (2012): 927-930.

[25] Sleep disturbance: Elizabeth M. Cespedes, Matthew W. Gillman, Ken Kleinman, Sheryl L. Rifas-Shiman, Susan Redline, and Elsie M. Taveras. Television Viewing, Bedroom Television, and Sleep Duration From Infancy to Mid-Childhood. Pediatrics, April 14, 2014.

[26] Diane Gilbert-Diamond, Zhigang Li, Anna M. Adachi-Mejia, Auden C. McClure, James D. Sargent. Association of a Television in the Bedroom With Increased Adiposity Gain in a Nationally Representative Sample of Children and Adolescents. JAMA Pediatrics, 2014; DOI: 10.1001/jamapediatrics.2013.3921

[27] Saunders, Lucinda E., et al. "What Are The Health Benefits Of

Active Travel? A Systematic Review Of Trials And Cohort Studies." Plos ONE 8.8 (2013): 1-13.

[28] Global Coalition on Aging. "Destination Healthy Aging: The Physical, Cognitive and Social Benefits of Travel" 2013.

[29] Gump, B.B., et al "Are Vacations Good For Your Health? The 9-Year Mortality Experience After The Multiple Risk.." Advances In Mind-Body Medicine 17.3 (2001): 201.

Community

[1] CDC. Chronic Disease and Health Promotion. Center for Disease Control and Prevention. 2012.
[2] Christakis, Nicholas A., and James H. Fowler. "The Spread Of Obesity In A Large Social Network Over 32 Years." New England Journal Of Medicine 357.4 (2007): 370-379.

[3] Hruschka, Daniel J., et al. "Shared Norms And Their Explanation For The Social Clustering Of Obesity." American Journal Of Public Health 101.S1 (2011): S295-S300.

[4] Robinson, Eric, et al. "What Everyone Else Is Eating: A Systematic Review And Meta-Analysis Of The Effect Of Informational Eating Norms On Eating Behavior." Journal Of The Academy Of Nutrition & Dietetics 114.3 (2014): 414-429.

[5] Jessica Gokee LaRose, Tricia M. Leahey, Brad M. Weinberg, Rajiv Kumar, Rena R. Wing. "Young adults' performance in a low intensity weight loss campaign." Obesity, 2012; DOI: 10.1038/oby.2012.30

[6] Ding, Eric, et al. "Microclinic Social Network Lifestyle Intervention for Weight Loss and Obesity Management: A 10-

Month Randomized Controlled Trial." Circulation.
2013; 127: A009

[7] Burke, Moira, et al. "Social network activity and social well-being." Proceedings of the SIGCHI Conference on Human Factors in Computing Systems. Pages 1909-1912
ACM New York, NY, USA 2010.

[8] Kross, Ethan, et al. "Facebook Use Predicts Declines In Subjective Well-Being In Young Adults." Plos ONE 8.8 (2013): 1-6.

[9] Sorkin, Dara, Karen S. Rook, and John L. Lu. "Loneliness, Lack Of Emotional Support, Lack Of Companionship, And The Likelihood Of Having A Heart Condition In An Elderly Sample." Annals Of Behavioral Medicine 24.4 (2002): 290.

[10] Jaremka, Lisa M., et al. "Loneliness Promotes Inflammation During Acute Stress." Psychological Science (Sage Publications Inc.) 24.7 (2013): 1089-1097.

[11] Jaremka, Lisa M., et al. "Loneliness Predicts Pain, Depression, And Fatigue: Understanding The Role Of Immune Dysregulation."Psychoneuroendocrinology 38.8 (2013): 1310-1317.

[12] Victor, Christina R., and Ann Bowling. "A Longitudinal Analysis Of Loneliness Among Older People In Great Britain." Journal Of Psychology 146.3 (2012): 313-331.

[13] Chi, Chiao, Weng Li-Jen, and Amanda L. Botticello. "Social Participation Reduces Depressive Symptoms Among Older Adults: An 18-Year Longitudinal Analysis In Taiwan." BMC Public Health 11.1 (2011): 292-300.

[14] Buettner, Dan. "Creating Communities (Blue Zones) That Enhance The Quality Of Life For Current And Future Generations." Nation's Cities Weekly 34.22 (2011): 5-7.

[15] Cohen, Sheldon, et al. "Sociability And Susceptibility To The Common Cold." Psychological Science (Wiley-Blackwell) 14.5 (2003): 389.

[16] Holt-Lunstad, Julianne, Timothy B. Smith, and J. Bradley Layton. "Social Relationships And Mortality Risk: A Meta-Analytic Review." Plos Medicine 7.7 (2010): 1-20.

[17] Savage, D.C. "Microbial ecology of the gastrointestinal tract." Annual Review of Microbiology. 1997. 31: 107-33.

[18] Ried, Kathryn. "Timing and intensity of light correlate with body weight in adults." PLoS ONE 9(4): e92251. doi:10.1371/journal.pone.0092251

[19] J. Thompson Coon, K. Boddy, K. Stein, R. Whear, J. Barton, M. H. Depledge. "Does Participating in Physical Activity in Outdoor Natural Environments Have a Greater Effect on Physical and Mental Wellbeing than Physical Activity Indoors? A Systematic Review." Environmental Science & Technology, 2011; 110203115102046 DOI: 10.1021/es102947t

[20] Miyazaki, Yoshifumi, et al. "Physiological benefits of forest environment: based on field research at 4 sites." Japanese Journal of Hygiene. 2011 Sep;66(4): 663-9.

[21] Miyazaki, Yoshifumi, et al. "Preventative medical effects of nature therapy." Japanese Journal of Hygiene. 2011 Sep;66(4): 651-6.

[22] Louv, Richard. "Children's Nature Deficit: What we know – and Don't know." Children & Nature Network. September 2009.

[23] Post, Stephen. "It's Good to Be Good: Science Says it's So." http://www.stonybrook.edu/bioethics/goodtobegood.pdf

[24] Hamilton, David. "Why Kindness is good for you." Hay House. 2010.

[25] James H. Fowler, and Nicholas A. Christakis. "Cooperative behavior cascades in human social networks." PNAS, March 8, 2010 DOI: 10.1073/pnas.0913149107

Love

[1] Chun Siong Soon, Marcel Brass, Hans-Jochen Heinze & John-Dylan Haynes. Unconscious determinants of free decisions in the human brain. Nature Neuroscience April 13th, 2008.

[2] University of Rochester. "Our Unconscious Brain Makes The Best Decisions Possible." ScienceDaily.

[3] Kelly K. Bost, Angela R. Wiley, Barbara Fiese, Amber Hammons, Brent McBride. Associations Between Adult Attachment Style, Emotion Regulation, and Preschool Children's Food Consumption. *Journal of Developmental & Behavioral Pediatrics*, 2014; 35 (1): 50 DOI:10.1097/01.DBP.0000439103.29889.18

[4] Chiang, Po-Huang, et al. "Bidirectionality And Gender Differences In Emotional Disturbance Associations With Obesity Among Taiwanese Schoolchildren." Research In Developmental Disabilities 34.10 (2013): 3504-3516.

[5] Wink, Paul. "George E. Vaillant, Triumphs Of Experience: The Men Of The Harvard Grant Study." Society 51.2 (2014): 184-187.

[6] M. Becker, et al. "Cultural Bases for Self-Evaluation: Seeing Oneself Positively in Different Cultural Contexts." Personality and Social Psychology Bulletin, 2014; DOI:10.1177/0146167214522836

[7] "Childhood Emotional Problems And Self-Perceptions Predict Weight Gain In A Longitudinal Regression Model." BMC Medicine 7.(2009): 46-54.

[8] Opperman, M. C., and H. E. Roets. "The Creation And Manifestation Of Reality Through The Re-Enactment Of Subconscious Conclusions And Decisions." Journal Of Heart-Centered Therapies 12.1 (2009): 3-98.

[9] Kraft, Tara L., and Sarah D. Pressman. "Grin And Bear It: The Influence Of Manipulated Facial Expression On The Stress Response." Psychological Science (Sage Publications Inc.) 23.11 (2012): 1372-1378.

[10] Sedikides, Constantine, et al. "Are Normal Narcissists Psychologically Healthy?: Self-Esteem Matters." Journal Of Personality & Social Psychology87.3 (2004): 400-416.

[11] Taylor, SE. "Illusion and well-being: A social psychological perspective on mental health." Psychology Bulletin. 1988. Mar 103 (2): 193-210.

[12] Fredrickson, Barbara L., et al. "Open Hearts Build Lives: Positive Emotions, Induced Through Loving-Kindness Meditation, Build Consequential Personal Resources." Journal Of Personality

& Social Psychology 95.5 (2008): 1045-1062.

[13] Terry, M, & Leary, M 2011, 'Self-compassion, self-regulation, and health', Self & Identity, 10, 3, pp. 352-362, Academic Search Complete, EBSCOhost, viewed 28 April 2014.

[14] Emmons, Robert A., and Robin Stern. "Gratitude As A Psychotherapeutic Intervention." Journal Of Clinical Psychology 69.8 (2013): 846-855.

[15] Hart, Jane. "Practicing Gratitude Linked To Better Health: A Discussion With Robert Emmons, Phd." Alternative & Complementary Therapies 19.6 (2013): 323-325.

[16] Almas, Alisa N., et al. "Effects Of Early Intervention And The Moderating Effects Of Brain Activity On Institutionalized Children's Social Skills At Age 8." Proceedings Of The National Academy Of Sciences Of The United States Of America (2012): 17228-17231.

[17] Grewen KM, Girdler SS, Amico J, et al. MD Effects of partner support on resting oxytocin, cortisol, norepinephrine, and blood pressure before and after warm partner contact. Psychosom Med. 2005;67:531-538.

[18] Light, Kathleen C., Karen M. Grewen, and Janet A. Amico. "More Frequent Partner Hugs And Higher Oxytocin Levels Are Linked To Lower Blood Pressure And Heart Rate In Premenopausal Women." Biological Psychology 69.1 (2005): 5-21.

Truly Sustainable Living

[1] Kopali, Albert. "Analysis Of The Sustainability Of Agricultural Farms Through Agri-Environmental Indicators At The Level Of Biodiversity And Landscape." Albanian Journal Of Agricultural Sciences 12.4 (2013): 539-544.

[2] Tilman, David. "Biodiversity & Environmental Sustainability Amid Human Domination Of Global Ecosystems." Daedalus 141.3 (2012): 108-120.

[3] University Of Minnesota. "Diversity Of Species Triumphs." Science Daily, 26 Oct. 2001.

[4] Howard, Richard D., J. Andrew DeWoody, and William M. Muir. "Transgenic Male Mating Advantage Provides Opportunity For Trojan Gene Effect In A Fish." Proceedings Of The National Academy Of Sciences Of The United States Of America 101.9 (2004): 2934-2938.

[5] Peekhaus, Wilhelm. "Primitive Accumulation And Enclosure Of The Commons: Genetically Engineered Seeds And Canadian Jurisprudence." Science & Society 75.4 (2011): 529-554.

[6] Peekhaus, Wilhelm. "Primitive Accumulation And Enclosure Of The Commons: Genetically Engineered Seeds And Canadian Jurisprudence." Science & Society 75.4 (2011): 529-554.

[7] Heeren, Gudrun A., Joanne Tyler, and Andrew Mandeya."Agricultural Chemical Exposures And Birth Defects In The Eastern Cape Province, South Africa A Case - Control Study." Environmental Health: A Global Access Science Source 2.(2003): 11-8.

[8] Weselak, Mandy, et al. "Pre- And Post-Conception Pesticide

Exposure And The Risk Of Birth Defects In An Ontario Farm Population." Reproductive Toxicology 25.4 (2008): 472-480.

[9] Khan, Dilshad et al. "Effect of Synthetic Pyrethroid Pesticide Exposure During Pregnancy on the Growth and Development of Infants" Asia Pac J Public Health July 1, 2013 25: 72S-79S

[10] Mansour, Sameeh A. "Pesticide Exposure—Egyptian Scene." Toxicology 198.1-3 (2004): 91-115.

[11] Eskenazi, Brenda, Asa Bradman, and Rosemary Castorina. "Exposures Of Children To Organophosphate Pesticides And Their Potential Adverse Health Effects." Environmental Health Perspectives Supplements 107.(1999): 409.

[12] Mostafalou, Sara, and Mohammad Abdollahi. "Pesticides And Human Chronic Diseases: Evidences, Mechanisms, And Perspectives." Toxicology & Applied Pharmacology 268.2 (2013): 157-177.

[13] Hayes, Tyrone B., et al. "Pesticide Mixtures, Endocrine Disruption, And Amphibian Declines: Are We Underestimating The Impact?." Environmental Health Perspectives 114. (2006): 40-50.

[14] Pettis, Jeffery S., et al. "Crop Pollination Exposes Honey Bees To Pesticides Which Alters Their Susceptibility To The Gut Pathogen Nosema Ceranae." Plos ONE 8.7 (2013): 1-9.

[15] Hackett, Kevin J. "Bee Benefits To Agriculture." Agricultural Research 52.3 (2004): 2.

[16] Marinari, Sara, et al. "Chemical And Biological Indicators Of Soil Quality In Organic And Conventional Farming Systems In Central Italy." Ecological Indicators 6.4 (2006): 701-711.

[17] Walsh, Bryan. "This Year's Gulf of Mexico Dead Zone Could be the Biggest on Record". Time. 2013.

[18] Birkhofer, Klaus, et al. "Long-Term Organic Farming Fosters Below And Aboveground Biota: Implications For Soil Quality, Biological Control And Productivity." Soil Biology & Biochemistry 40.9 (2008): 2297-2308.

[19] Shuman, M and Hoffer, D. 2007. "Leakage Analysis of the Martha's Vineyard Economy: Increasing Prosperity through Greater Self-Reliance." (Training and Development Corporation).

[20] Swenson, D. 2009. "Investigating the Potential Economic Impacts of Local Foods for Southeast Iowa." Ames, IA: Iowa State University. (Leopold Center for Sustainable Agriculture).

[21] Goetz, Stephan J., and Hema Swaminathan. "Wal-Mart And County-Wide Poverty." Social Science Quarterly (Wiley-Blackwell) 87.2 (2006): 211-226.

[22] Wagstaff, Adam. "Poverty And Health Sector Inequalities." Bulletin Of The World Health Organization 80.2 (2002): 97.

[23] "Does Poverty Predispose To Obesity?" Nutrition Today 39.1 (2004): 17.

[24] Drewnowski, Adam. "Poverty and obesity: The role of energy density and energy costs". American Journal of Clinical Nutrition. January 2004. Vol 79. no. 1 (6-16).

[25] Drewnowski, Adam. "Does social class predict diet quality?". American Journal of Clinical Nutrition. May 2008. vol 87. no 5 (1107-1117).

[26] Chupeau, Yves and Vaucheret, Herve. "Ingested plant miRNAs regulate gene expression in animals". Cell Research (2012) 22:3-5. Doi:10.1038/cr.2011.164

[27] LeBlanc et al. Formation of Hydroxymethylfurfural in Domestic High-Fructose Corn Syrup and Its Toxicity to the Honey Bee (Apis mellifera). Journal of Agricultural and Food Chemistry, 2009; 57 (16): 7369

[28] Meunier, Julien, et al. "Birth And Expression Evolution Of Mammalian Microrna Genes." Genome Research 23.1 (2013): 34-45.

[29] Zierath, Juleen. "Acute exercise remodels promoter methylation in human skeletal muscle". Cell Metabolism. Volume 15, Issue 3, 405-411

[30] Allgayer, Hubert, et al. "Short-Term Moderate Exercise Programs Reduce Oxidative DNA Damage As Determined By High-Performance Liquid Chromatography-Electrospray Ionization-Mass Spectrometry In Patients With Colorectal Carcinoma Following Primary Treatment." Scandinavian Journal Of Gastroenterology 43.8 (2008): 971-978.

[31] Nicole D. Powell, Erica K. Sloan, Michael T. Bailey, Jesusa M. G. Arevalo, Gregory E. Miller, Edith Chen, Michael S. Kobor, Brenda F. Reader, John F. Sheridan, and Steven W. Cole. "Social stress up-regulates inflammatory gene expression in the leukocyte transcriptome via β-adrenergic induction of myelopoiesis". PNAS 2013 110: 16574-16579.

[32] Jia, Yimin, et al. "Maternal Low-Protein Diet Affects Epigenetic Regulation Of Hepatic Mitochondrial DNA Transcription In A Sex-Specific Manner In Newborn Piglets Associated With GR Binding To Its Promoter." Plos ONE 8.5 (2013): 1-9.

[33] Dominguez-Salas, Paula. "Maternal nutrition at conception modulates DNA methylation of human metastable epialleles." Nature Communications. 5:3746, 2014.

[34] Lambrot, R. "Low paternal dietary folate alters the mouse sperm epigenome and is associated with negative pregnancy outcomes". Nat Communications. Vol 4 (2013): No 2889. doi:10.1038/ncomms3889

[35] Drake, Amanda J., et al. "An Unbalanced Maternal Diet In Pregnancy Associates With Offspring Epigenetic Changes In Genes Controlling Glucocorticoid Action And Foetal Growth." Clinical Endocrinology 77.6 (2012): 808-815.

[36] Hackett, Jamie A., et al. "Germline DNA Demethylation Dynamics And Imprint Erasure Through 5-Hydroxymethylcytosine." Science 339.6118 (2013): 448-452.

[37] Coghlan, Andy. "Genes marked by stress make grandchildren mentally ill". NewScientist. 03 Nov 2010. Issue 2785.

[38] Hurley, Dan. "Trait Vs Fate." Discover 34.4 (2013): 48-55.

[39] Kaiser Family Foundation. Health Care Costs: A Primer. Published May 2012.

CPSIA information can be obtained
at www.ICGtesting.com
Printed in the USA
LVOW10s1532020217
523022LV00011B/873/P